TABLE OF CONTENTS

SPECIAL PRAYER

Special thanks for God's unconditional blessings because without him there could be no me. Father, I come to you today grateful, I come to you hopeful and humble, I come to you a new man of purpose.

I thank you father for the many blessings you've given me such as my family and rejuvenated health. I thank you for blessing my wife Pastor Mary Kearney, she's my spiritual advisor, editor, and the Creative Director of "All About Entertainment 156" &

"Boom in Your Face" podcast for helping me with my book. I thank you for blessing the Doctors at Celebration Bariatric Center Dr Smith, Cathy and all the nurses that you've anointed to work through their hands, father I ask that you bless this book and everyone that reads it may it bring them comfort and strength to push forward.

Father, I ask that you give them peace in knowing that with faith, their blessings will follow. Father, I ask for blessings to those struggling with obesity and all the illness that comes with it.

Father, we know that you are the great I am. Always able and willing to fix things and that with you all things are possible! Father, I thank you for your mighty hands of healing and ask that you continue to bless me in my process and all those who are needing and willing to accept your terms for your, Blessings!

Amen!

Acknowledgments

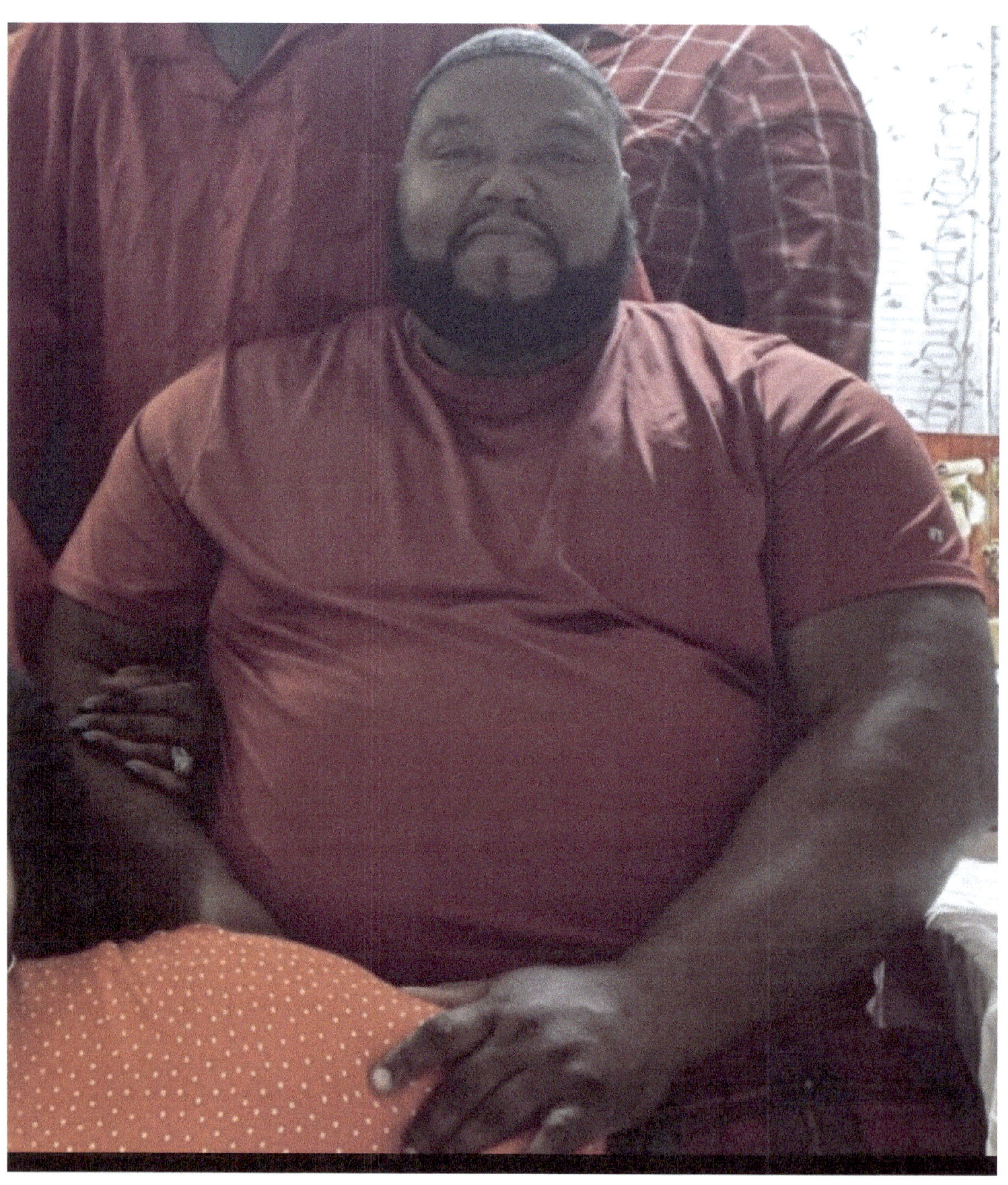

BARIATRIC

SURGERY

&

SPIRITUALITY

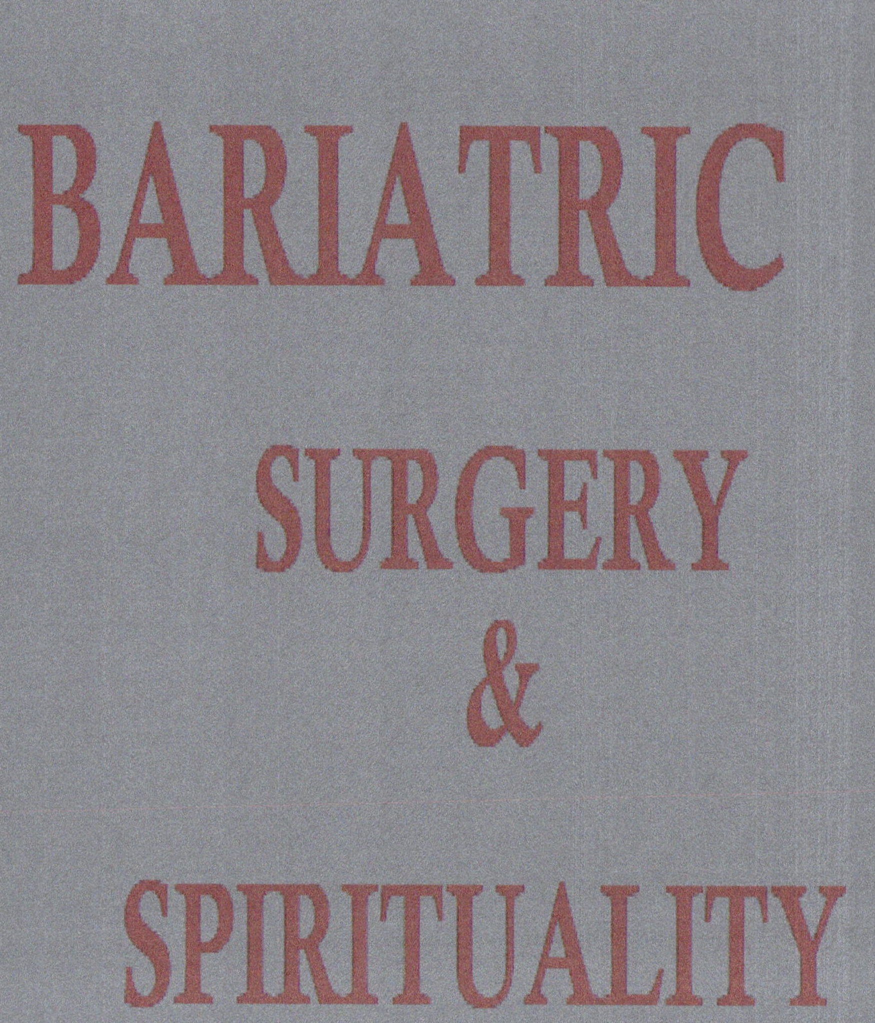

BY JAMES KEARNEY

Acknowledgements

Special Thanks to my beautiful wife Pastor Mary

Kearney for her support with dealing with my

illnesses, issues, and obesity over the years. For

over 30 years she has been and continues to be the

love of my life and has been supportive,

inspirational, caring, and very instrumental to the

successes in my life.

My wife Pastor Kearney has given me everything in my life that's important and meaningful to becoming a successful man.

She has provided a loving home for our family and has guided my five beautiful and accomplished children. She has prayed for me to have drive to be the best man that is pleasing unto our creator. She has willed and inspired me the strength to live through my darkest struggles.

I'd also like to thank my five amazing children for their support and their consistent help and thoughtfulness over the years dealing with my illnesses, issues, and obesity. Thanks to my eldest son James Kearney II for his struggles with me in my weight loss journey, going to the gym and running with me he's an awesome young man.

He's played four years of college football and is one of the smartest men that I know on earth thank you James Kearney II. I'd also like to thank my eldest daughter Doreen she's outstanding; she's blessed me with my one grandson Nigel who's incredibly important to me, a future NFL player!

My daughter Jessica, and sons Jaysson, and Little Jay for always supporting their father in anything I wanted to do, most of all being patient with my health.

I want to thank my mother Mary and father John Henry Hicks for assuring that I was born. I also want to thank my friends and family that have allowed me to vent and gave me input on my decision. And, lastly to my Walmart pharmacy family in Kissimmee

for making things easy and stress free during my

healing process.

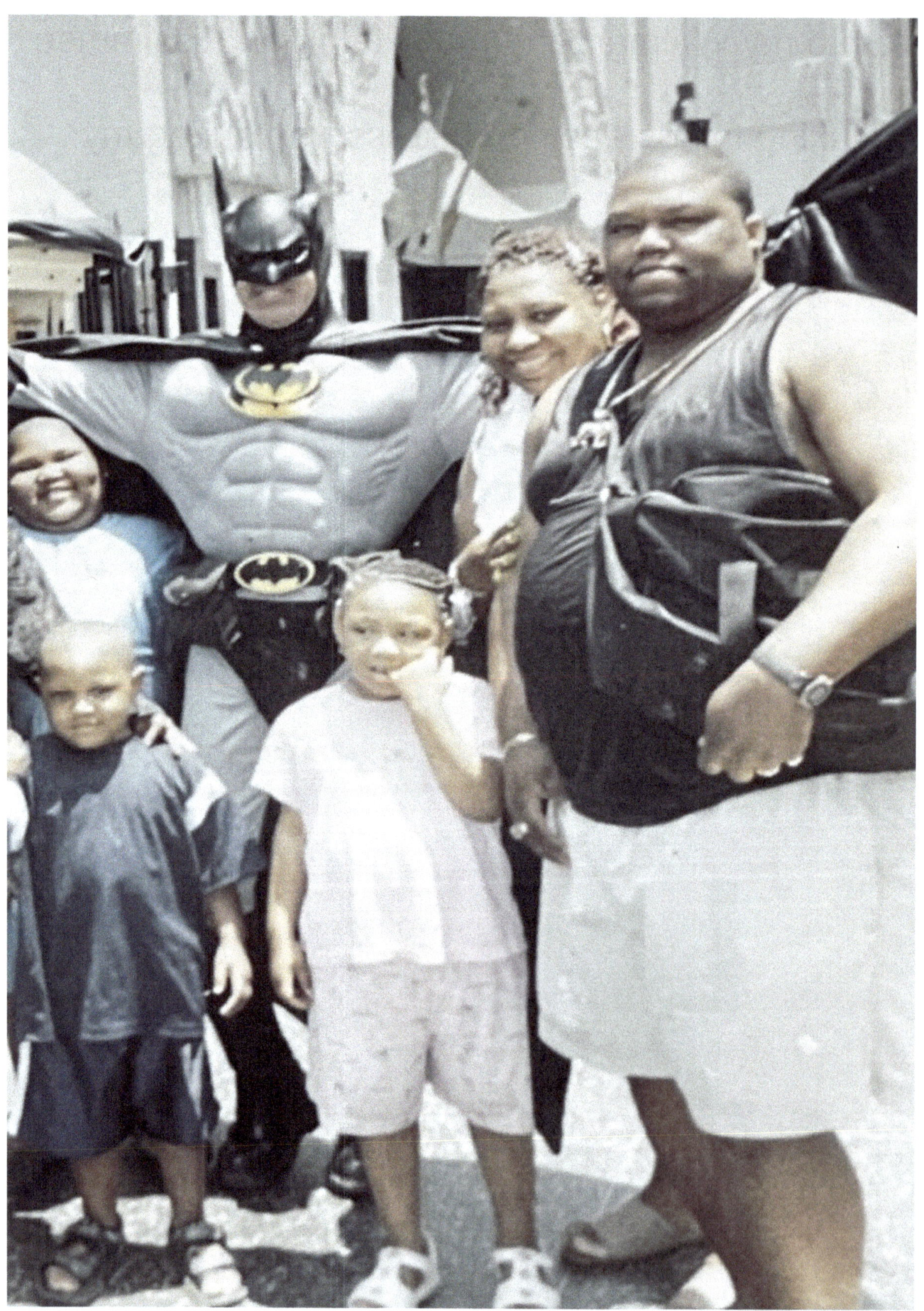

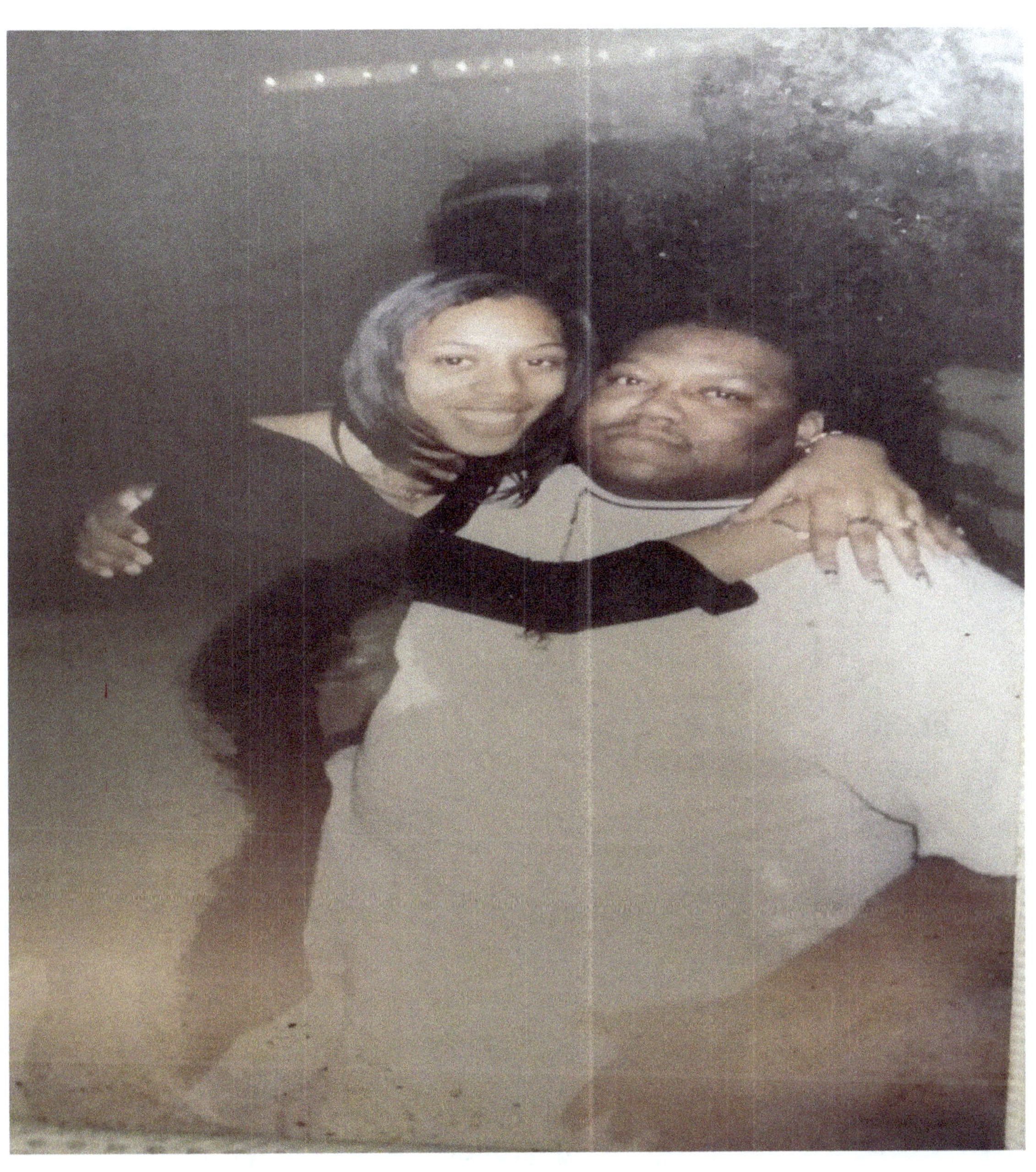

Type of Surgery

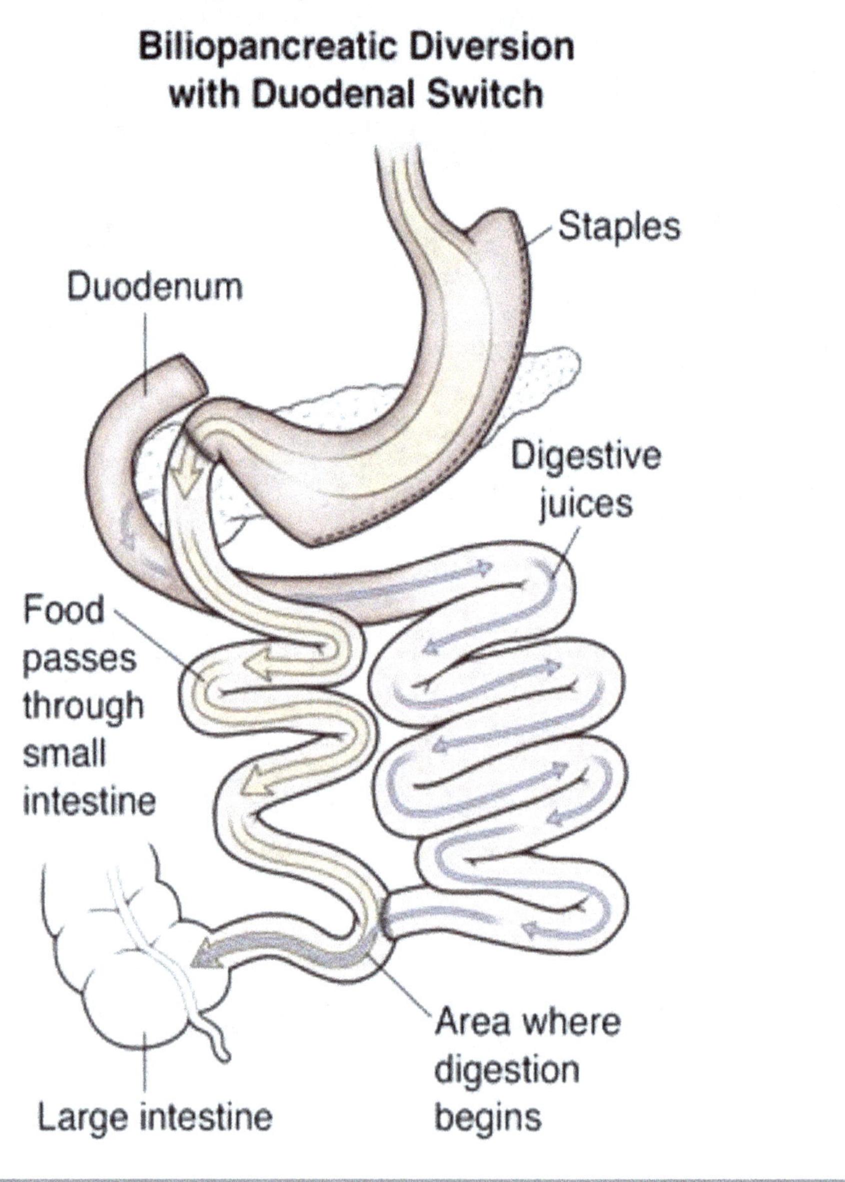

INTRODUCTION

Hello, this book is about Bariatric Surgery and Spirituality, and how it has saved my life and continues, too. Are you a great candidate for Bariatric Surgery? Are you tired of people telling you that all you need to do is exercise more and eat less? Well, the fact is that until you feel better it's hard to do better. Your Health plays a major role in the conditioning of your body so first we need to work on feeling better.

My name is James Kearney, and, in this book, you'll

find out if it's for you or not and I'll be discussing the

good, the bad, and the truth about Bariatric Surgery

and Spirituality from the standpoint of a patient.

CHAPTER ONE

LIFE CHANGE FOR

BETTER HEALTH

There are several different types of bariatric surgeries. You should meet with your physician to decide which one is best for you. In this book I'll be talking about the Duodenal Switch (DS). Are you a great candidate for Bariatric Surgery?

Currently, only 34% of Florida adults are at a healthy weight, approximately 28% are obese, and about 36% are overweight. On our current trend, there is a high probability that by 2030, the proportion of Florida adults at a healthy weight will reach only 30%. This is according to the Florida

Department of Health. In this book I'll be talking

about the Duodenal Switch (DS), better known as

the DS Switch.

The DS Switch is a weight-loss surgery designed to

treat people who have severe obesity. It combines a

sleeve gastrectomy with an intestinal bypass. The

DS Switch is the most complicated but also the most

effective bariatric surgery.

It's especially effective for patients with type 2

diabetes. The DS Switch is a weight-loss operation

that modifies your stomach and your small intestine. It combines a gastrectomy (removal of part of your stomach) with an intestinal bypass, which makes the path your food takes through your intestines shorter. This restricts how much food your stomach can hold, and how much nutrition your small intestine can absorb from your food.

(This makes it a "malabsorptive" procedure). It also reduces the hunger hormones that your stomach and small intestine normally produce. Your healthcare provider may recommend bariatric surgery if you have clinically severe obesity (class III), which means you're at high risk of or are already experiencing obesity-related diseases.

These include metabolic syndromes such as high blood pressure, high cholesterol, and high blood sugar, which are precursors to heart disease, kidney disease and diabetes. Cardiovascular disease: hypertension, arterial disease, vascular disease, heart attack, stroke. Respiratory diseases: asthma, obstructive sleep apnea, obesity hypoventilation syndrome. Metabolic diseases: hyperlipidemia,

insulin resistance and diabetes.

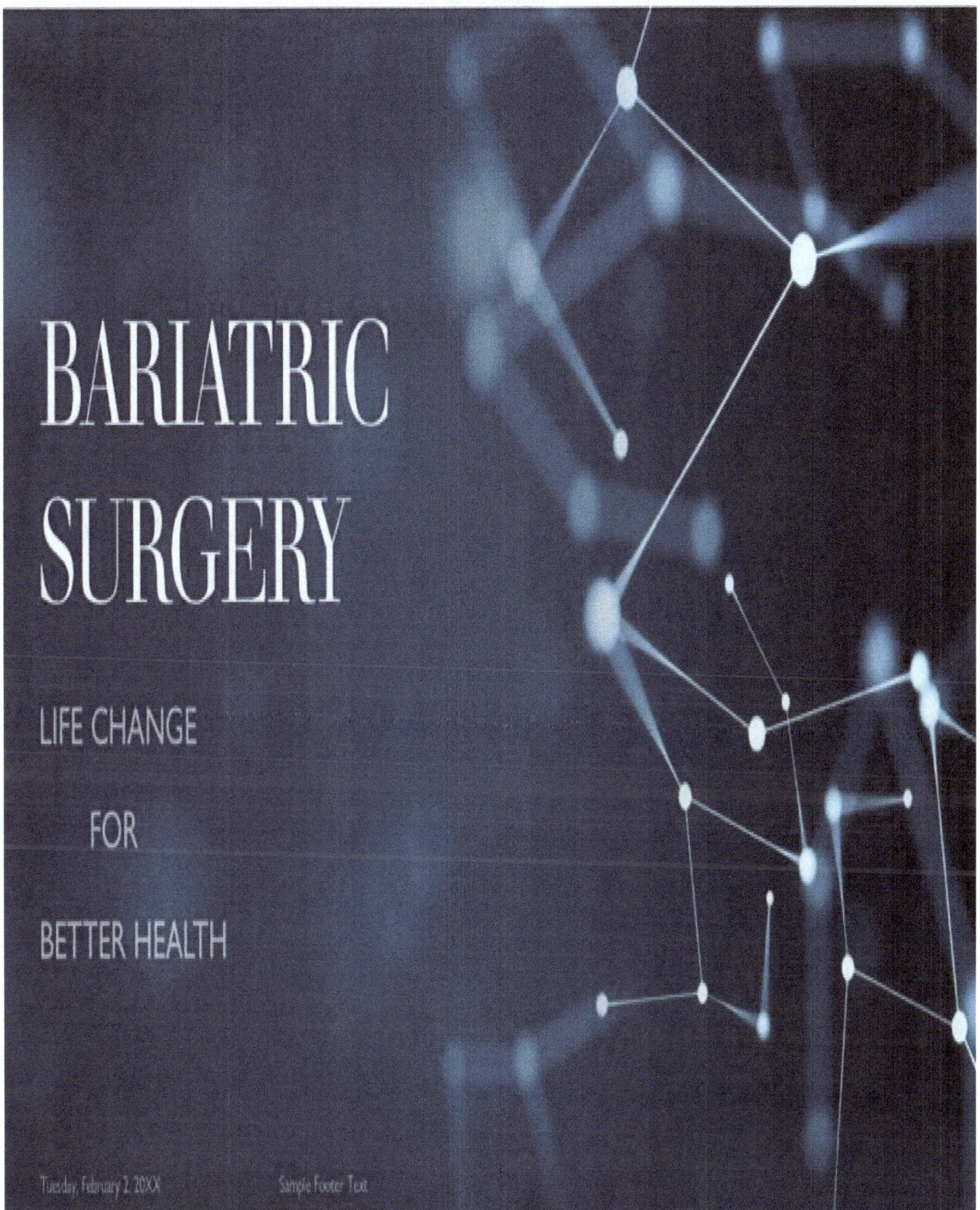

BARIATRIC SURGERY
LIFE CHANGE
FOR
BETTER HEALTH
Tuesday, February 2, 20XX
Sample Footer Text

Gastrointestinal diseases: non-alcoholic fatty liver

disease, nonalcoholic steatohepatitis. Reproductive

diseases: polycystic ovary syndrome, infertility.

Musculoskeletal pain: back strain, weight-bearing

osteoarthritis.

Cancer: especially colorectal cancer and liver

cancer. You may be diagnosed with class III obesity

if you have a BMI of 40 or higher, or if you have a

BMI of 35 and one of these related diseases. The

DS Switch is less commonly performed than other

bariatric surgeries because it is more complicated and extreme.

It involves more cutting and stitching in your digestive system and takes out or bypasses more of your gastrointestinal tract than other procedures do. This makes it riskier for complications, both during the procedure and afterwards. The DS Switch reduces the absorption of essential vitamins and minerals that can result in serious, long-term complications.

Some people that have the DS Switch may develop anemia, osteoporosis, or kidney stones. In addition, some people who have undergone the DS Switch procedure are at high risk for calcium and iron deficiencies. This group of people are also at high risk for deficiencies in vitamins A, D, E, and K, the fat-soluble vitamins.

Although, rare a thiamine deficiency can sometimes happen after DS surgery. This can damage the nervous system if untreated. Up to 18% of people with a DS Switch surgery also develop some element of protein-energy malnutrition.

When severe, this condition is known as kwashiorkor, a severe and potentially life-threatening form of malnutrition. It's a must after having this surgery to have blood work done every three months. This will let you know what vitamins you need. I've had to add several new vitamins to my system.

If you have DS Switch surgery, you will need to take vitamin and mineral supplements and have regular blood testing for the rest of your life. This is done to prevent severe vitamin deficiencies and related complications. Even if you take the supplements as

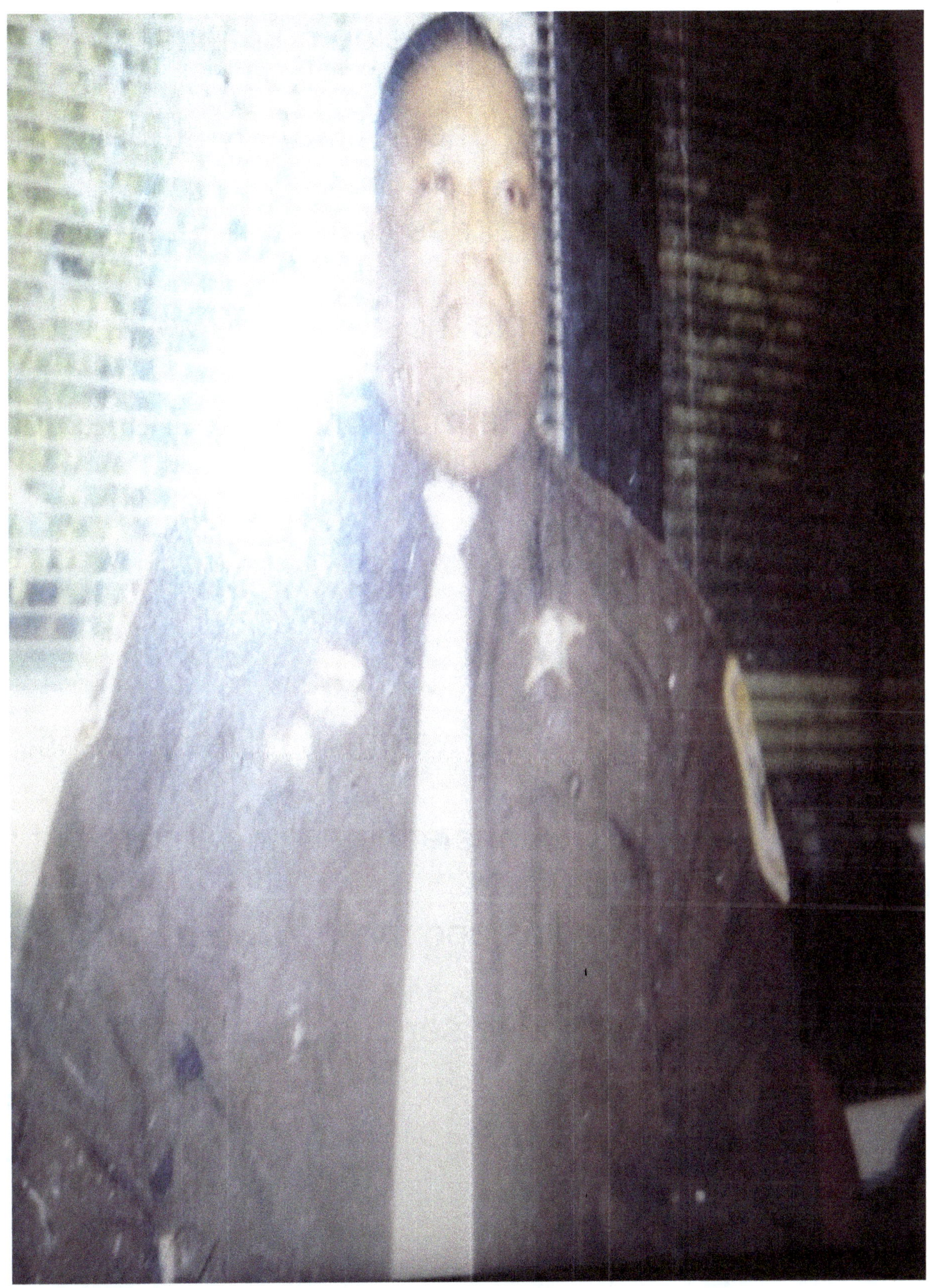

prescribed, you still may develop nutritional problems and need treatment. Like any surgery, the DS Switch procedure carries certain risks: However, the DS Switch is also the most effective weight-loss surgery method, with the most profound and lasting results.

We don't all start out overweight, but life happens. Some of us were previous athletes or dancers but as we get older our bodies and the way we burn calories change. If you're serious about getting your life back and taking a stand to be healthy then

maybe this surgery is for you.

All surgeries are dangerous and come with risks like

death or serious complications. Know your facts and

don't be discouraged your health is very important to

yourself and family.

CHAPTER TWO
THE BEGINNING

Six months ago, I set out on a journey to regain my life back I was scared, I was confused, I didn't know what to expect. I discussed this surgery with my wife and children some gave good feedback; some gave negative feedback. Once my mind was set and I decided to go along with the surgery, I tried to stay away from all the negative talk.

You must take into consideration your family's opinion but understand you must live in your body and if you're on a bad path with your health maybe it's time for a change. The only way to succeed with

this type of surgery is to have your loved ones that

bring positive vibes to you, and an incredible

surgeon and bariatric team!

Having people that you trust and love around you is

very important because you will need them in some

form or fashion. Before, after, and during the surgery

your team matters. You will be tested mentally and

physically stay tough you can do it!

A life's change is coming soon! You'll have to see many doctors and go through many clearances but stay strong and look to the future of regaining your life back. I cannot say this will be an easy road because it's not but if you're committed to feeling better and being better there's no stopping your possibilities.

NEGATIVITY

No one wants to be looked at in a negative way. No one wants to be embarrassed or ashamed of themselves because they've gained a little weight over the years. If you've felt any of these types of emotions, you might what to consider thinking about having this specific surgery.

The decision is yours and <u>yours alone</u>. Don't allow anyone to force your decision. Take your time to think about it, meditate about it, and most importantly pray about it!

I set out on a journey about six months ago to change my life. I was determined and undeterred about my decision and knew I had to move forward.

I won't lie, it's a very hard and difficult road but that's

why having your faith is crucial. Continue reading

this book and you might find a positive outcome!

To start off with some insurance companies might

mandate that you have 6-months of a physician

supervised dieting. Your family physician can

oversee your supervised medical diet which would

include a weigh-in once a month and consultation.

You will also have several appointments scheduled

for you from your bariatric clinic.

Some may include cardiologist, nephrologist, and lots of blood work depending on your medical history. This is all necessary to make sure that you have a safe and successful surgery.

My advice is that you do your research on who will be performing your surgery because your life is in their hands. Also, do the research on the hospital you will do your recovery in because they will be the first people to take care of you after surgery.

After the dieting for six months and all the different

hoops you must jump through, hopefully you can be

scheduled for your surgery. You must lose a certain

amount of weight before you can be scheduled for

your surgery this will be set by your surgeon. After

losing some weight you may have second thoughts

but stay strong.

These surgeries are in high demand so you may

have to wait another month or two or three hopefully

not that long but who knows. If you opted to pay

without insurance, you'll still have to see a few doctors, but the process will be faster.

The day had come that I'd received a phone call from my bariatric clinic to schedule my surgery, now all those tough nerves I once had are all gone. As my stomach rumbles and eyes tear, my heart aches because I don't know what to expect.

It's important to have your family members support your Health decision. Talk to them, they will help you more than anything. This is a big and life changing moment for me and my family. Weighing close to 400 pounds, I had refused to live like this any longer. I could hardly walk to the corner. I was always eating and always hungry never fully satisfied.

I suffered with different ailments for nearly 20+ years, high blood pressure, high cholesterol, diabetes, asthma, and back & knee pain. I was taking hands full of pills everyday just to survive through until the next day.

This was not working out for me, and I had enough!

The medication made me even sicker, so they

added more medication to offset the previous

sickness.

Some of My Actual Medications

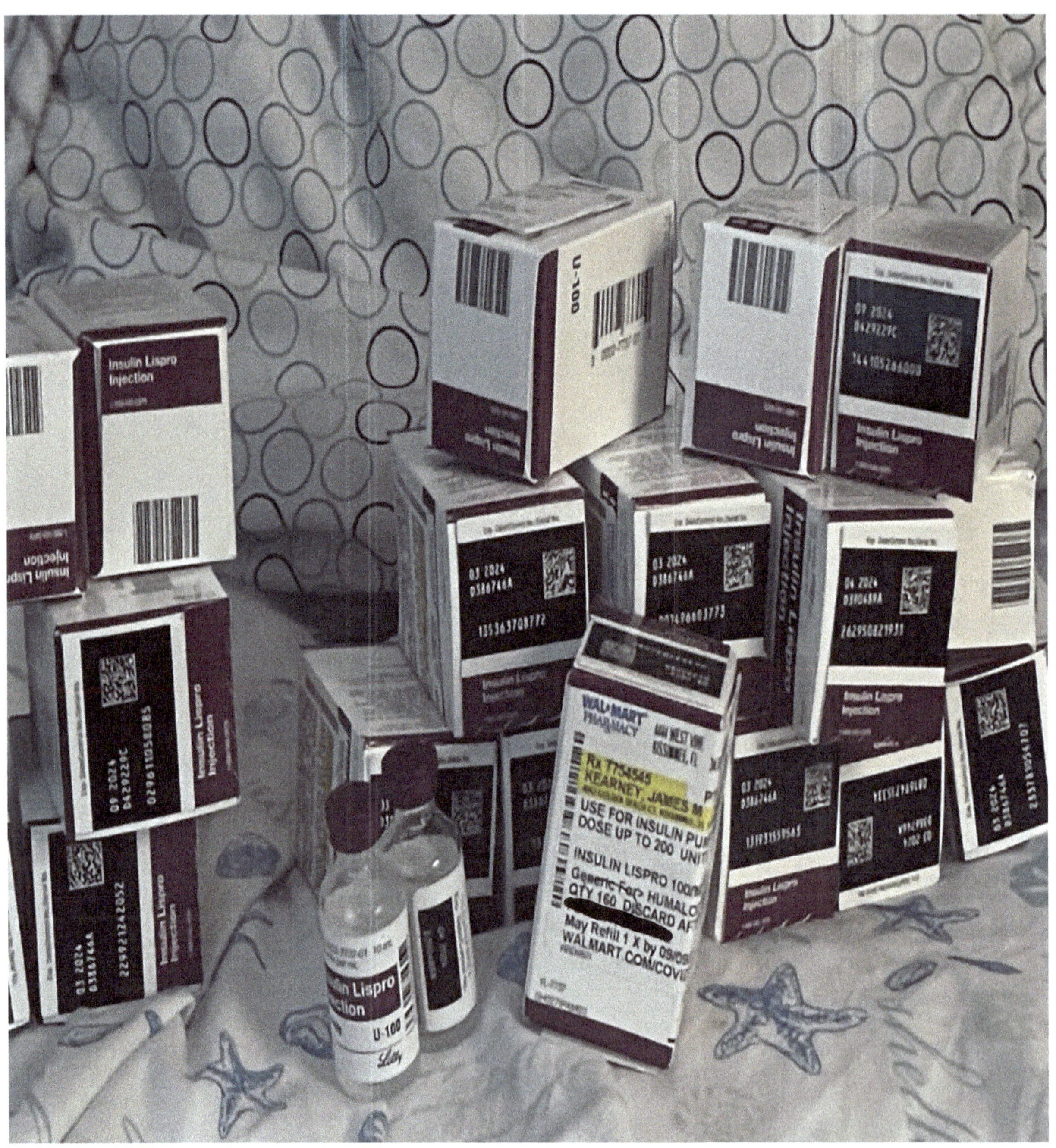

Medicine	Dose
EXAMPLE: *Aspirin*	*325 mg*
Asprin	325
Invokana	300
Clonidine	0.2
Zafirlukast	20
Isosorb mono	20
Furosemide	40
Hydralazine	100
Clonazepam	0.5
Tizanidine	4
Topiramate	50
Lyrica	100
Amlodipine	5
Sinvastatin	40
Colchicine	0.5
Hydrocyzine	50
Lisinopril	40
Metoprolol	100
Butal	50-321-40
Humalog	100
Ocxy	15
Testosterone get	1.62
Budesonide inhalation	0.5
Proair	
Allopurinol	300
Diclofenac	3%
Sumatriptan	50

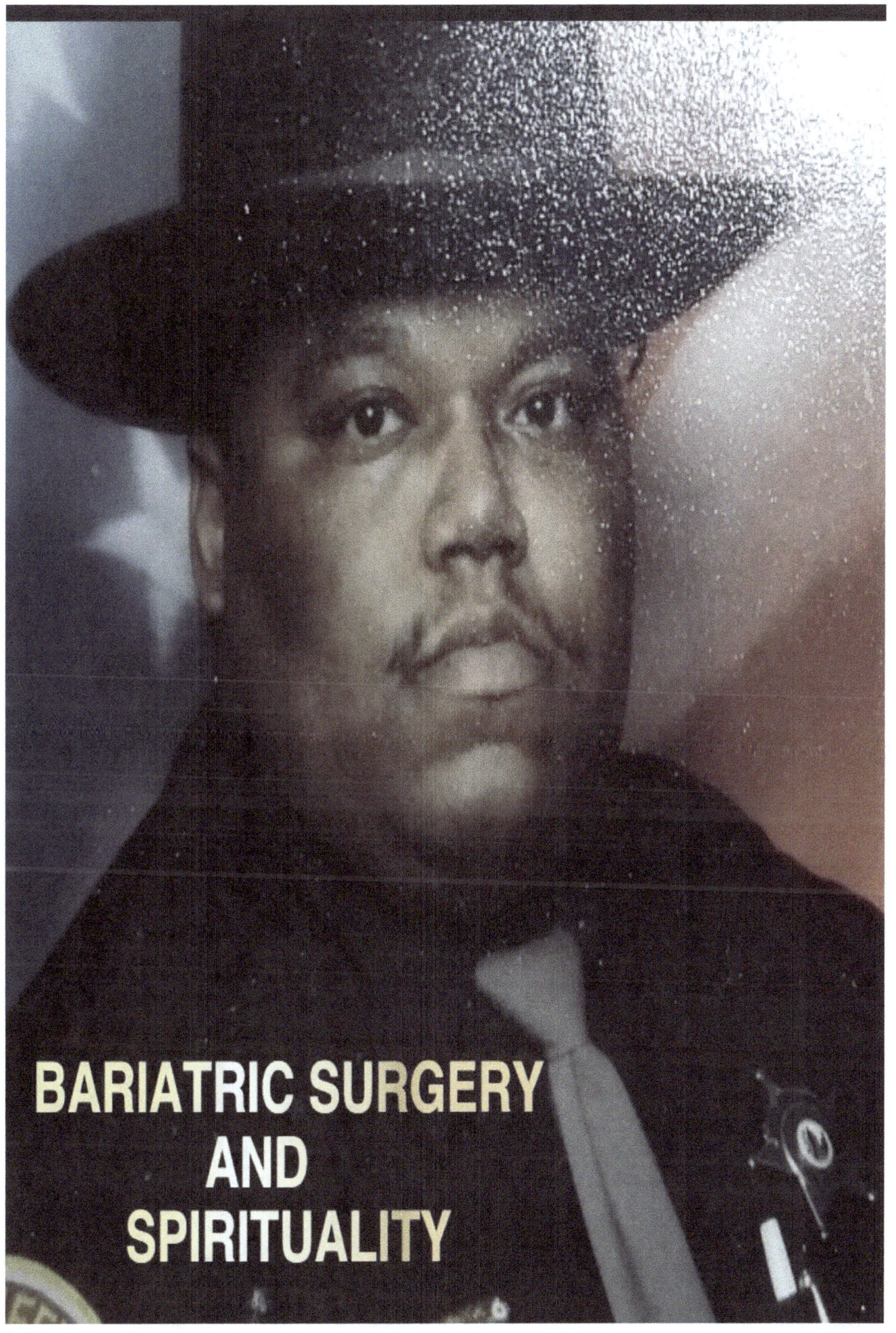

BARIATRIC SURGERY
AND
SPIRITUALITY

CHAPTER THREE

CHANGE

Today's the big day I have no idea what to expect other than the information given to me by the bariatric center. I have no idea if I will make it through surgery. I'm fearful but with God and my family I had the courage to proceed with the surgery.

I remember going into a waiting room with my wife, she prayed over me for the Lord's grace and mercy. Then, shortly after that she kissed me and went to the waiting area. I had no idea if I would ever see her again.

The last thing I do remembered was talking to my surgeon and the anesthesiologist. When I woke up from the surgery and it was over, I remember feeling tremendous pain in my abdomen from the surgery. I felt like a part of my body was missing and it was.

THE STRUGGLE

A good Bariatric clinic will provide every and all information pertaining your surgery. Things like; what to expect before the surgery and what to expect after the surgery down to the tee. They will also make sure that you have time to purchase all your items to make things easier after surgery like 2oz cups and hot thermal cups.

After surgery, I was brought to a hospital ward that specializes in the care of bariatric surgical patients.

Within hours the medical staff in the hospital had me up and walking around the hospital. I remember being so excited to see my wife and family during this time.

I wanted to know if I had done the right thing with making the right decisions for my life. Because this decision will not only affect you but each one of your family members that you live with and love. I had to consider the main person that it would affect which is my life's partner my wife!

My body was so badly beaten over the years from the abuse of my behaviors. Some caused by myself from overeating and over drinking, gorging myself till I was overly stuffed. I was on an insulin pump for many years and taking lots of medication three times a day in the form of pills.

Walking settles your bowels and at first, you'll feel very clumsy, very awkward, and your equilibrium will be off. Keep walking as much as possible things will get better.

Sleepy Bowels

I'm sure the hospital was specific with their instructions when I was discharged my memory was a little foggy from the meds. I remember having my wife escort me downstairs from the hospital when it was time for discharge. I was so excited to go home but the pain didn't get better.

In fact, it got worse when I got home, I continued to take my medication which was a lot of pills for blood pressure, high cholesterol, asthma, Gouty arthritis, and diabetes. I didn't realize I was supposed to pace myself with taking my medication one pill every twenty minutes. A few days went by, and I was starting to feel extreme pain. I was back in the hospital two days later due to my bowels not moving.

I want to be clear this surgery deals with your intestines predominantly so there are some narcotics that are not allowed. During surgery they'll put your intestines to sleep, and after surgery they must awaken your intestines back up. Sometimes it may take longer for some people to jump start there intestines back to functioning normally again.

In my case the surgeon had to go back in to clean up some scare tissue. After the second surgery I was taken back up to the bariatric floor were the medical staff provided superb service to me. They were encouraging me and made sure that I was up and walking and moving around.

Narcotics will slow this process down so be prepared to go through some of the pain without pain medication. I stayed in the hospital for close to two weeks the second time dealing with pain and learning about my new pouch. Not able to take anything in liquid or food of any sort.

After seven or eight days they decided to give me liquid nourishment and the fear arose in me once again. A special team was brought up with a machine to x-ray my arm so they could insert a pic in my arm. I was terrified because they explain to me the many possibilities of things that could go wrong with this pic.

However, I knew my body needed the nourishment, so I proceeded with the procedure. The pharmacy in the hospital prepared a special cocktail for me made up based on my daily blood work with detailed nourishment needs.

It was in a large bag, white, and creamy like coconut milk. These bags would supply my body with nutrients over the next few days. Before that I had what the staff calls a banana bag running through my IV.

The medical staff was outstanding as they came and did my vitals, talked with me when my family wasn't there, and they kept me sane while I was in the hospital. Time is ticking as the days went by my children had planned a 30-year anniversary for myself and my wife. I was fearful that I would never make this beautiful event that was planned for us.

I've never spoken to God as much as I did in this moment. I don't know how religious you are, but religion plays a big role when you make life decisions. As I prayed, I asked God to heal me to take the pain away so I may be released in time to enjoy my 30th anniversary with my beautiful wife and children.

The next day came, and the surgeon came to see me he said, "we're going to try you on liquids for a day or two and see how that works". I explained to him that I was trying to leave the hospital because my anniversary was coming up. However, being a very professional physician, he explained to me how serious he was about me getting better, feeling better, and succeeding with the surgery.

Being patient was helpful because the next day the nurses reported that I was taking the liquids well and soon I would be going home. I knew I had to stay another day now that the doctor wanted to see how well I took in liquid protein. It was hard at first, but I continued to sip so I could get out the hospital. The next day the report came back that I was able to take in the liquid protein so finally the doctor said, "OKAY, I'm going to release you now".

Excited and overwhelmed with happiness that I was going home but I wanted to feel better. I wanted to be able to dance with my wife. I wanted to enjoy my family. It was a scary time for me, but God made sure that all my prayers were answered, and I was returning home.

A couple of days before my big anniversary event I tried to feel better, but the surgery changed my sense of smell. Everything smelt bad things like people, food, and soaps would upset my senses. The sound of people would annoy me, and I didn't want to be bothered with anyone. I didn't want anyone to be concerned about me and the transition I was going through. I forced myself to get dressed and put on a

fake smile for appearances. Forcing myself to have

fun that really wasn't fun for me at all!

JAMES & PASTOR MARY'S FAMILY

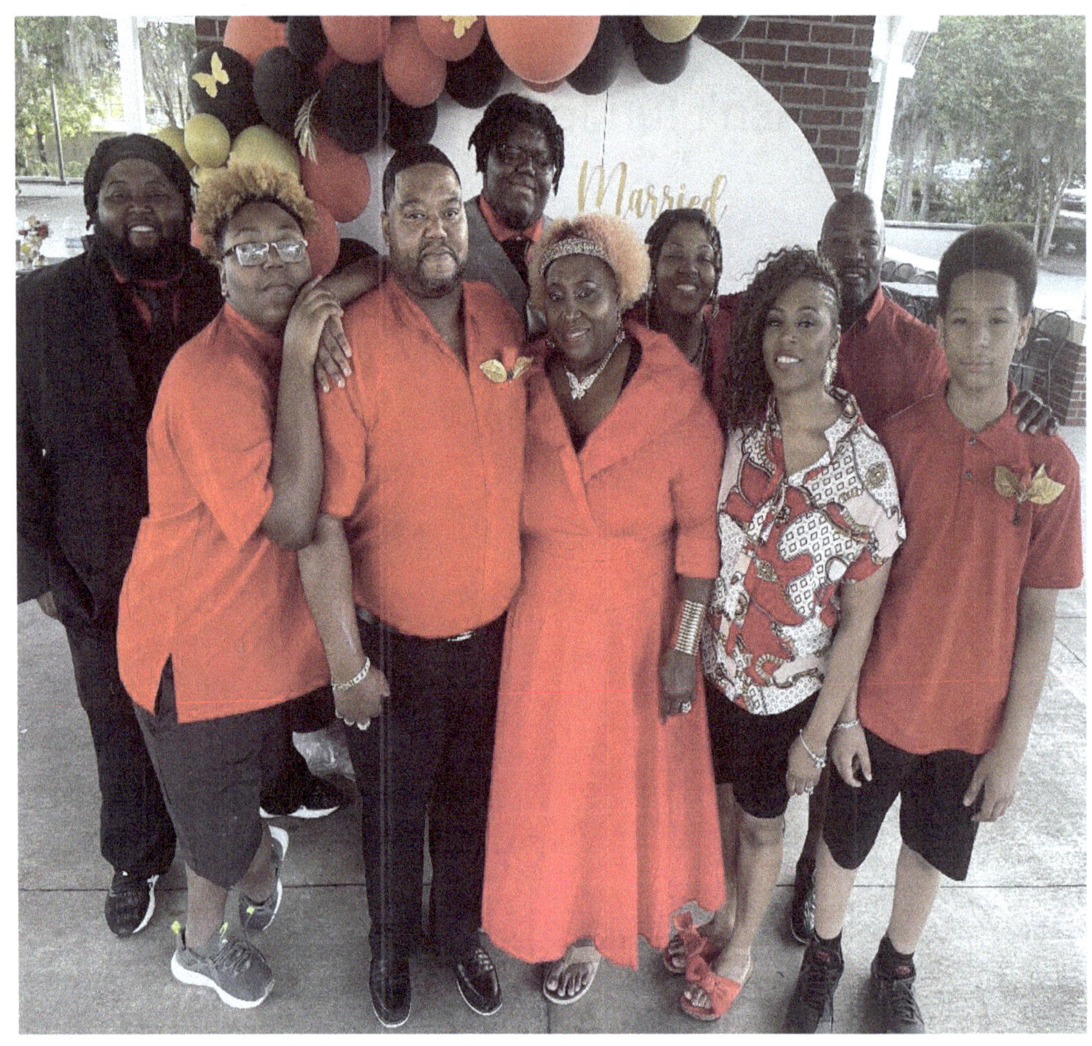

30TH ANNIVERSARY

CHAPTER FOUR

AFTER SURGERY BLUES

I never knew things would be this hard. I never knew that each pill that you took you had to wait 15 to 20 minutes to take the next one and that's not fun when you're doing 10 pills three times a day. Do the math, that's a long time and a lot of sipping. It was just hard work and even harder work ahead.

Everything I wanted to do became very difficult and a hard task. Smelling certain foods would trigger my appetite but as my stomach would start to rumble desiring the food not being able to consume the food was torturous to me. At first, I didn't know why I was hungry. I didn't know why I was having these feelings and thoughts about food. I knew I couldn't change everybody else's diet in the household, so I had to change my response.

One thing that affects me and my wife the most is the extremely smelly GAS and the loud rumbling in my stomach (Lol)! It is so bad that I must run out the room every time I have to pass gas. I did not want my wife to have to suffer. However, the stool that I now pass smells even worse than the gas that I silently release.

I'm sure it's the high protein diet that I'm on causing the fragrant aroma.

There will also be some nauseating times, but you can do it. I'll suggest that you stock up on <u>Gas-X</u>! Never give up, keep pushing you will have a lot to deal with, but your health is the most important thing in the world to you and your family. I decided to love myself a little more and be thankful for the body and soul that was given to me.

Wanting to enjoy life a little more, wanting to share life with my family, and loved ones a little longer. No one is born perfect, so you must take care of the body you have to the best of your ability.

NEW DAY

Better days are coming but hard work is ahead. I never thought that hot broth would be so good. I can remember my 1st cup of soup that my wife made me it was some chicken stock with low sodium it was amazing to me.

I couldn't take much but I took what I could and the warmth from the soup seemed to have comforted me. Your bariatric clinic will give you a specific amount of liquids you need to take every day and a specific number of proteins you need to take in every day.

They'll also advise you on stages of food that you can eat. By that I mean liquids and different stages of solid foods.

All this information will be provided to you by your Bariatric clinic. I didn't do well with the beginning phases of pain but as the pain started to subside my mind and stomach wanted to eat food again. Testing the waters and jumping over stages is never a good thing to do trust me you will pay the price!

Your pouch is too small and sensitive for complicated foods to break down. Overfilling this pouch can be very discomforting, feelings like heartburn on steroids, feelings like stabbing pain shooting through your heart. It will only take a few times for this to happen before your mind triggers and says, "Hey, I remember what happened last time I ate that". Or you'll drink too fast and severe pain will be the result. You'll get the message very fast, don't worry pain will train you.

As the days go by, and I go through the stages of food cycles, I struggle to meet my quota of liquids. A month goes by and I'm now able to meet my quota of liquids and wanting to eat certain foods but incapable of it. I decided to stick close to the diets that were provided for me from the Bariatric clinic.

My diet consists of lots of yogurt, protein shakes, green vegetables, and lots, and lots of water. I lost roughly 50 pounds while I was in the hospital, I was so excited about that. However, I was a little discouraged after three months that I hadn't lost any more weight. I was doing everything right and wondering why I am not losing weight.

Within the fourth month the scale started dropping and with every pound lost I gained energy and strength. I was able to walk more and become more active. I decided that I would include going to the gym three times a week and walking 2 miles a day but the 2 miles a day didn't work out as well as I thought.

My knees were hurting so I decided to do 2 miles every other day which worked out better for me. Now

I'm losing weight two sizes smaller. Feeling amazing and blessed, I can't stay out the mirror! Never knew what determination and hard work could do. As, the weight continues to fall off the better I feel. Guess I will be buying some new clothes very soon! Lol.

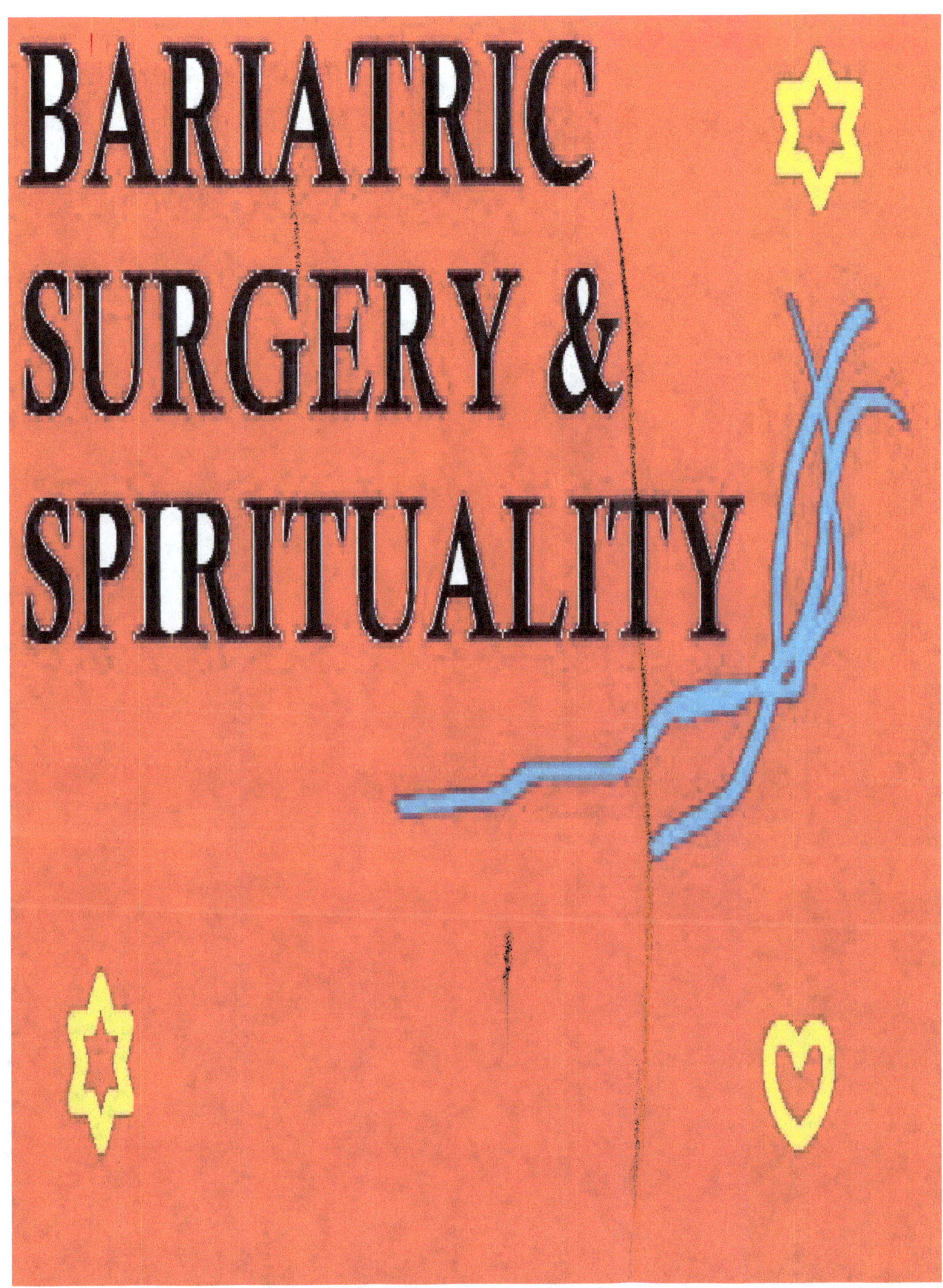

BARIATRIC
SURGERY &
SPIRITUALITY

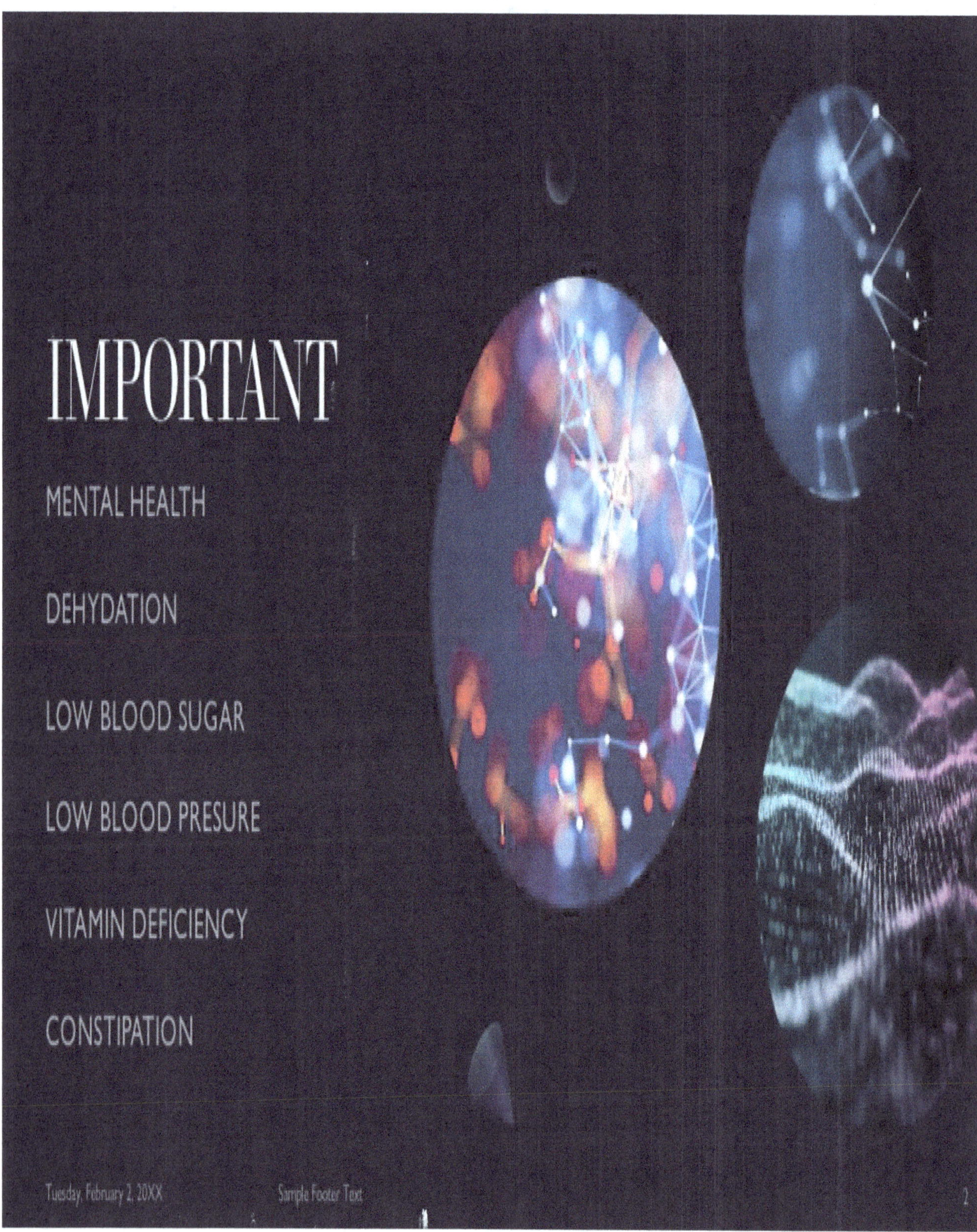

IMPORTANT
MENTAL HEALTH
DEHYDATION
LOW BLOOD SUGAR
LOW BLOOD PRESURE
VITAMIN DEFICIENCY
CONSTIPATION
Tuesday, February 2, 20XX
Sample Footer Text
2

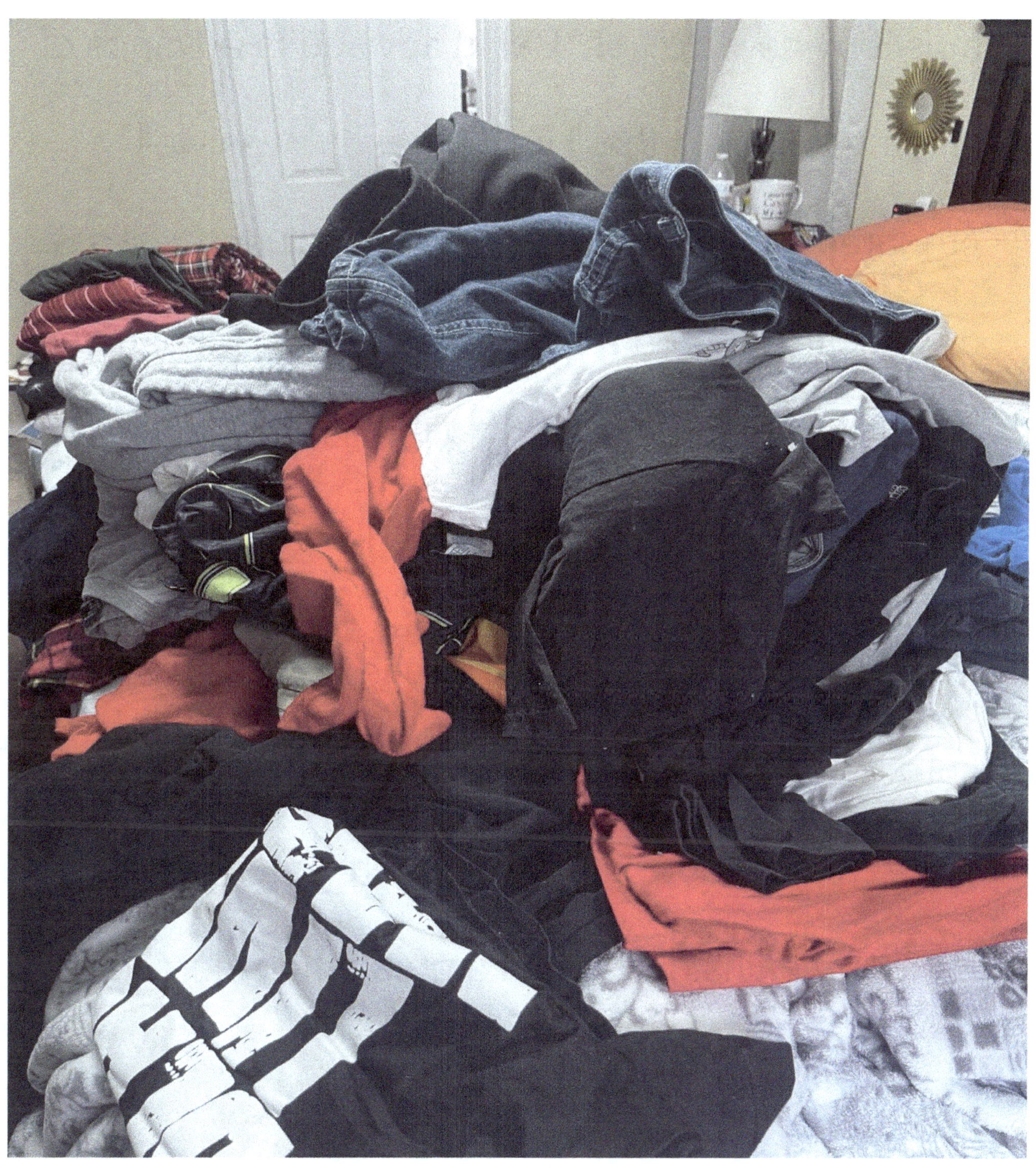

I'm excited but all my clothes are falling off me, so I must buy new clothes. Being advised in advance of different supplies that I would need; I was well prepared over the six months that included a scale, diabetic tester, and a blood pressure cuff. I had cups to keep my liquids warm or cold.

In the Fourth month, I had my check up with my surgeon. My blood work was drawn in advance and my A-1C was now 5.3 and I haven't been on insulin for four months. I also had a great cholesterol level and my kidney function improved.

I was excited because before surgery my best A1C was 7.3 that was with an insulin pump and now I'm testing in the normal ranges. The pump that I wore was every day, all day, all night, 24 hours a day with nonstop beeping of alarms. Warning if your blood sugar is going up or if your blood sugar is going down. After, a few years that can play a psychological game with your mind. It also affects your spouse sense of peace.

Still in the fourth month, I awakened with a very low blood pressure. I called my family physician and scheduled an appointment and he decided to start taking me off some of my blood pressure medications. I was overwhelmed with joy from hearing the new plan!

Having to take five different blood pressure pills three times a day is a very saddening experience to go through daily.

Now that I'm down to three blood pressure pills and no cholesterol pills, I'm starting to see more of the pros of my decision. In the beginning I was concerned if I was making the right decision or not. I felt that I made a mistake.

I felt like my life was over and then I asked God to please help me, please heal me, and strengthen my spirit & faith. There's no way to explain the thoughts that rolls through your mind when you're hurting and not knowing what to expect.

Now it's five months and all the pain has gone. My body has healed well and is still healing. But I know that if I had to do it again I would without a doubt. I feel unbelievable and unreal. Is this true?

Sometimes, I wake up and feel like it's a dream. I feel so amazing after feeling so sick and down for over 25 years. Some days I didn't even leave the bed. Hard work is still ahead!

There is no easy quick fix and if you're not willing to put in the time & work, don't do the surgery, it's not for you. Some people just think because they had the surgery they can sit around and do nothing. Well, let me tell you that's a bad mistake it will slow down your process!

After, going through such an intense surgery, you'll want to make the best of it. Now you'll start to remember old sayings like "No pain, no gain", and "Hard work pays off!". I'm here to tell you that my life has changed.

I'm so grateful to God first, my wife, my children, then my surgeon, and the entire staff. Not wanting to have another surgery I'm working hard to tighten my skin as the fat burns away. It will leave behind what you have stretched over the years dealing with obesity.

Now at the beginning of the 5th month I've noticed just how overstuffed I've been. Depending on your weight loss you will have to deal with sagging skin on different parts of your body. I personally use all kinds of products to deal with that issue. There are skin tightening creams you can rub on to help with that problem.

My favorite product to use is the sweat vest it's a special tank top that makes me sweat. Then, I put my waist trainer over that, then I start walking in the hot sun for 2 to 3 miles. Don't forget to put sunblock on (Lol). We can never get back to 21 but we can improve our chances to live longer and stronger.

I haven't run in over 35yrs for enjoyment. When I was a high school football star nicknamed Rock I'd loved running, I played the running back on the team, and the noise guard.

BARIATRIC SURGERY AND SPIRITUALITY

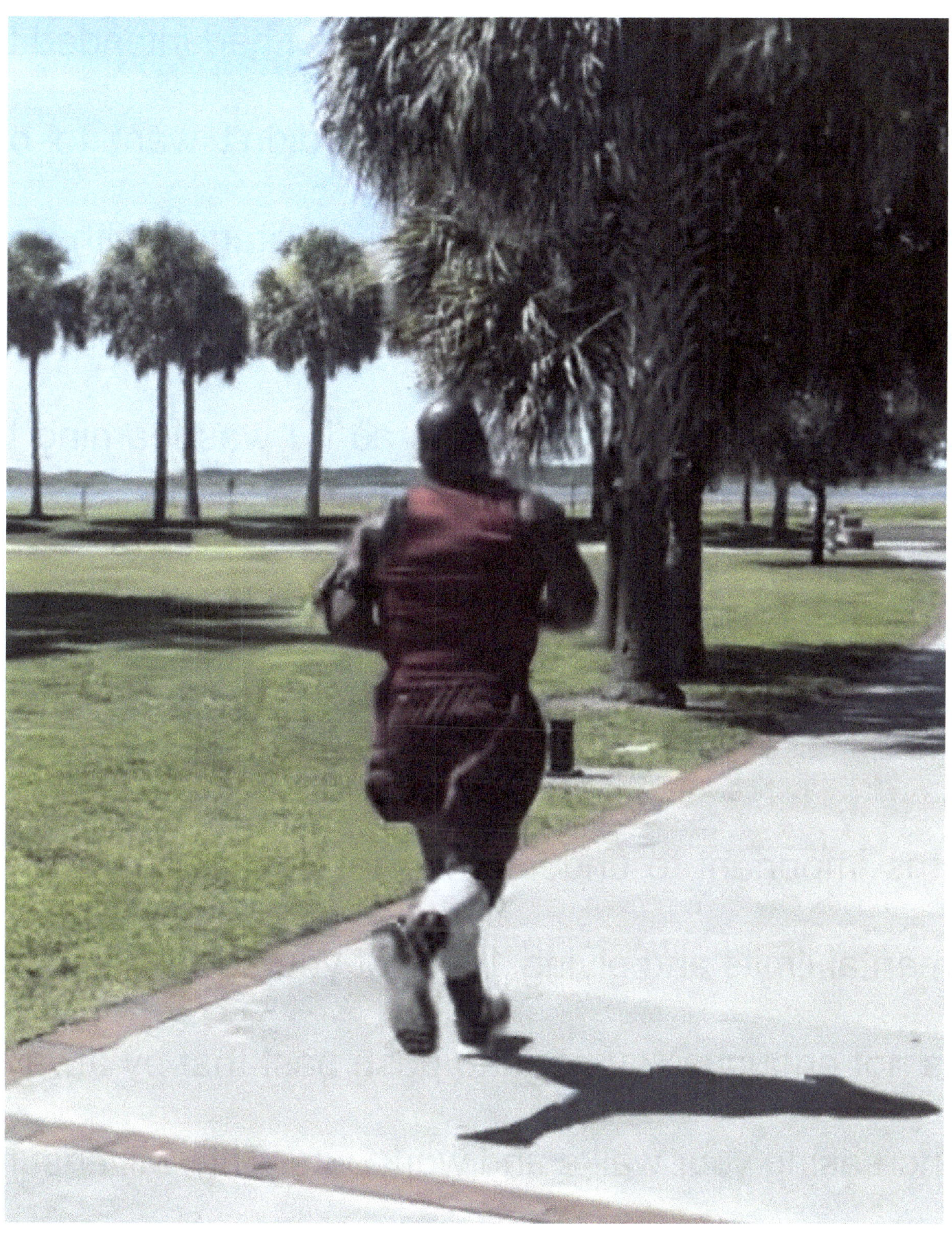

Today has brought new challenges I had intended to run again, but I was terrified. I didn't want to be humiliated trying to run in public. I started with one foot at a time then a slow jog wasn't too far behind, and it felt so amazing! It was as if I was learning to run again but I was determined not to let my fear stop me.

It is important to understand that pushing past your mental limits and giving 100% of yourself sometimes is not enough. You need to push past that by always increasing your walks and work outs. This will ensure true progress, while overcoming barriers that lie in the back of your mind. You will then start to see the true potential in your body.

When making your decision on the type of bariatric surgery it's best for you to talk to your doctor. I chose the DS switch because it seemed suitable for me. The DS switch has great success of patients not regaining their weight back. The way my body now processes food, I will no longer need insulin.

I will do everything in my power never to fall back into that self-forced situation again. Learning to live again: wow not being awakened by the screeching sound of beeps that my insulin pump would alert! What a blessing it is, a gift from God no matter what religion.

It is important to strengthen your spirituality during this time he is always listening and always healing. You so badly need this relationship right now! Some people Don't like to bring spirituality and science together in the same sentence. However, my take on that is one cannot exist without the other.

God anoints the doctors, surgeons, and nurses the same way he anoints a person to become a minister to work for him. This process is difficult and without my faith and belief in God there's no way I would've done the surgery. There's absolutely no way I could just trust my life to man alone.

What are your expectations of life? How do you perceive your future? Are you looking for healing in your soul? Are you looking for healing in your body? Are you looking for healing in your mind? Through science many things that weren't possible are now made possible but keep in mind someone overseas this progress as we travel through this world.

It's a journey some get it, and some don't, but at some point, in your life you will learn that there is a God no matter what religion you are, we all agree that there's a higher being. At some point you may have to fall to your knees and pray, Amen.

On the 4th of July months since my surgery, I'm feeling great. I'm enjoying the holiday like never before, appreciating all my blessings. It's pool time with the family and enjoying the aroma wafting from the grill.

Continuing my journey, I push forward practicing new great habits! It's important that you know your body. I find myself moving around so much more that sometimes I forget to take in my protein or drink my water. Do your best to try to remember!

CHAPTER FIVE

DANGERS

Today I'm lightheaded knowing my body I go test my

blood sugar, and it's 77 and dropping fast. Hmm?

Never thought I'd see the day when my blood sugar

dropped this low without insulin. You will get

incredible results if you put the work in.

What drove me crazy was listening to people say oh

you just need to work out, move more then you eat,

well until you feel better it's hard to do better. No

more bedtime during the day I want to indulge in life.

Another hurdle today I did my first sit-up without

assistance my stomach was so badly stretched and

so big I was unable to do sit-ups. My daily struggle for a new life continues as the temperatures reaches the triple digits. I'm unwilling to slow down; I'm moving forward with my daily activities. Today, I've jogged a little and walked a lot and when I was finished, I felt a little strange?

My head was dizzy, my mouth was dry, and I had the worst headache. My workout had caused me some tremendous sweating. Not being able to get enough liquids into my system to prevent dehydration I was feeling ill.

My wife had warned me that I probably was dehydrated and to seek some medical attention. That's when I knew it was really time to call the doctor! Most Bariatric clinics have a designated area for infusions be aware of the symptoms of dehydration. It's very important for you at those moments to know your new body and understanding your new body's alarm system.

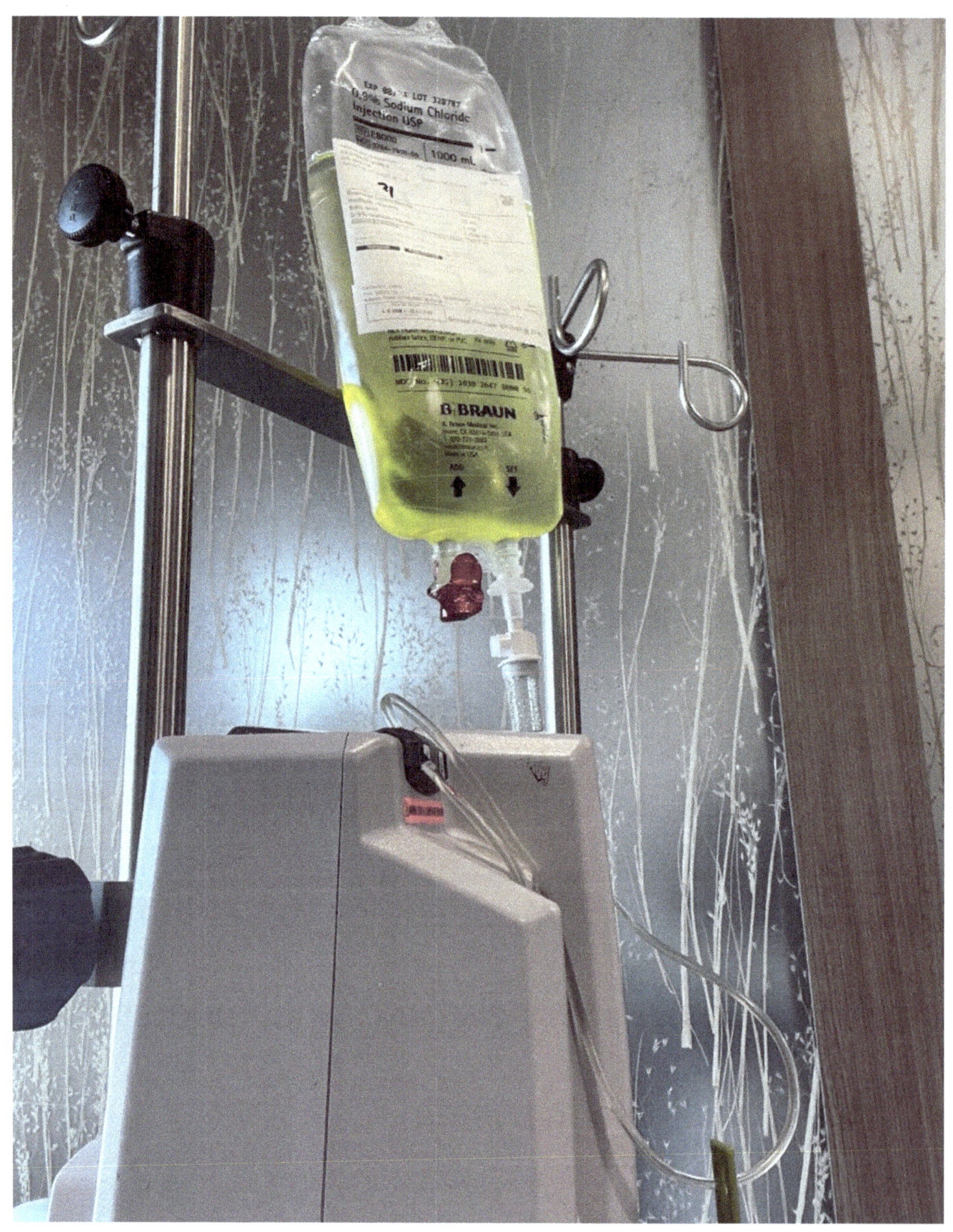

EXP 00x x LOT 328787
0.9% Sodium Chloride
Injection USP
1000 mL
B BRAUN
ADD   SET

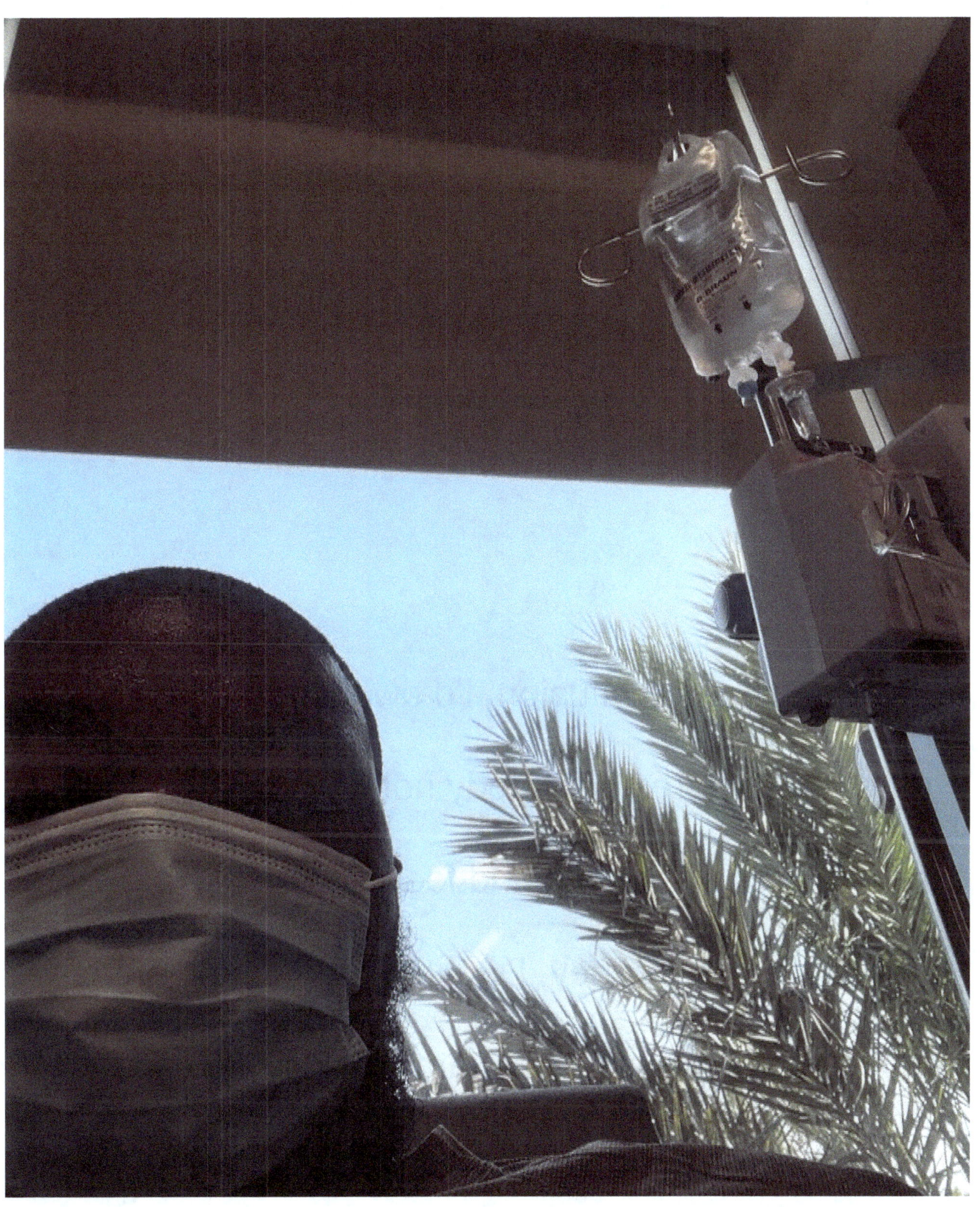

Don't struggle! Dehydration can be deadly and knowing the signs may save your life. Today, I find myself at the infusion center receiving fluids and nourishment through an IV-line. This infusion is a lengthy process of about 5 hrs.

The day after the infusion, I'd awakened to a refreshed and restored body not having any dehydration symptoms and feeling better.

Continuing my journey, I woke up today and started doing my daily weigh-ins. I am officially 120 pounds smaller than I was at my highest weight. I know I've spoken to you about the positive things connected with this surgery.

Now I'm going to share with you some things that may not be as positive to you and it will become a challenge. Being 120 pounds smaller I've received certain hints from my family that I'm too skinny. Now I'm too small and almost the smallest person in the house and sometimes it makes me feel not so good about the new look.

I'm also experiencing a reaction from my wife of over 30 years because when you go on this journey you don't just affect yourself, but you'll affect your spouse and everyone around you. My wife has been loving me for over 30 plus years and 25 of those years I've been over 350 pounds, so she's used to loving & accepting that big jolly guy.

Now I'm filling some distance between us, so I asked her if she was not happy about my weight loss? I feel like you are treating me a certain way and she said to me you must give me time to adjust to your new body because it's a rapid weight loss process and I'm just not used to this new look.

As we laid in the bed, I asked my wife to lay in my arms and when she did, she didn't get that same old soft cushion that she's been used to having. She said, "Wow! Where did you go!" Well, that made me feel awful and I'd explained to her how it made me feel and why it had made me feel that way.

Please make sure that your mental health status is in order because this surgery will test you mentally and physically. You'll deal with all types of challenges from dehydration to not getting enough nutrients. Even different reactions from your family members and loved ones.

People that have known you over the years as a big person will now look at you differently. As I fall to my knees, I pray to God to bring understanding into my family's life so that they may know that the surgery was necessary for me to move forward as a healthy person.

I'm the same person inside, my hearts the same, my soul is the same, but my physical appearance is under new construction. As the days grow closer to my 6-month recovery mark I'm able to enjoy food again just not as much at one time.

Continuing my journey, I find myself struggling to stay hydrated going through hot summer days. So, I decided to investigate different hydration powders and I ran across a couple of good ones.

I can't stress how important It is to stay hydrated during this time, as you work out you perspire but you're not able to take in copious amounts of liquids at one time. Therefore, you become susceptible to dehydration.

I hope this book brings comfort to your heart and eases the stress in your mind that with God and the proper doctors you will succeed in whatever it is you want to do. This is not an easy process so be prepared to work, and work, and work!

Now, instead of living to eat you will have to eat to live. As an older man I did not enjoy losing my hair it was very depressing to me there are so many effects of this surgery that can bring you down but with faith and trust you will get through it.

Somedays, I'm completely stressed trying to get enough liquids in to meet the daily requirements. This surgery is life changing it will change the way you think and change the way you live. Today at 5 months post-surgery I'm no longer on blood pressure medication or high cholesterol medication and my A1-C IS 5. I want to stress to you, "Please don't think that you can just have the surgery sit back and watch the miracle unfold because that is not the way the process works".

CHAPTER SIX
WHAT MADE ME DO IT

My day starts with a prayer and ends with a prayer. There is no right or wrong way to pray. He hears all and knows all for without him there would be no life and no world to enjoy.

I have always felt a burning deep inside my heart when I hear or read the words. I don't know if that's my calling to be a minister but when or if the time comes God will let me know.

My wife and oldest son are both ministers and very intelligent Godly people. When I pray I thank God first, then my wife, then my children. I want to live a long and healthy life so I can enjoy my grandkids and great grandkids one day. Life is not guaranteed to anyone, but you can live a healthy life, and a life that's full of joy and love.

Some people can stick to a diet and commit to a healthy lifestyle, but most of us struggle. Every day grinds gets to us. Working hard every day, family stress, and bills are some reasons we don't take proper care of ourselves. In a rush! Grabbing that fast food, not getting medical checkups.

This is how we begin to damage ourselves {SELF NEGLECT}. One illness leads to another illness, one medication leads to the next and before you know it you have 10 different prescription and you're now fighting for your life.

High Blood Pressure, Diabetes, and High Cholesterol these are some of the first signs that we are going in the wrong direction. It's not too late! You can reverse this; surgery is one option but if your strong enough you can fix this on your own.

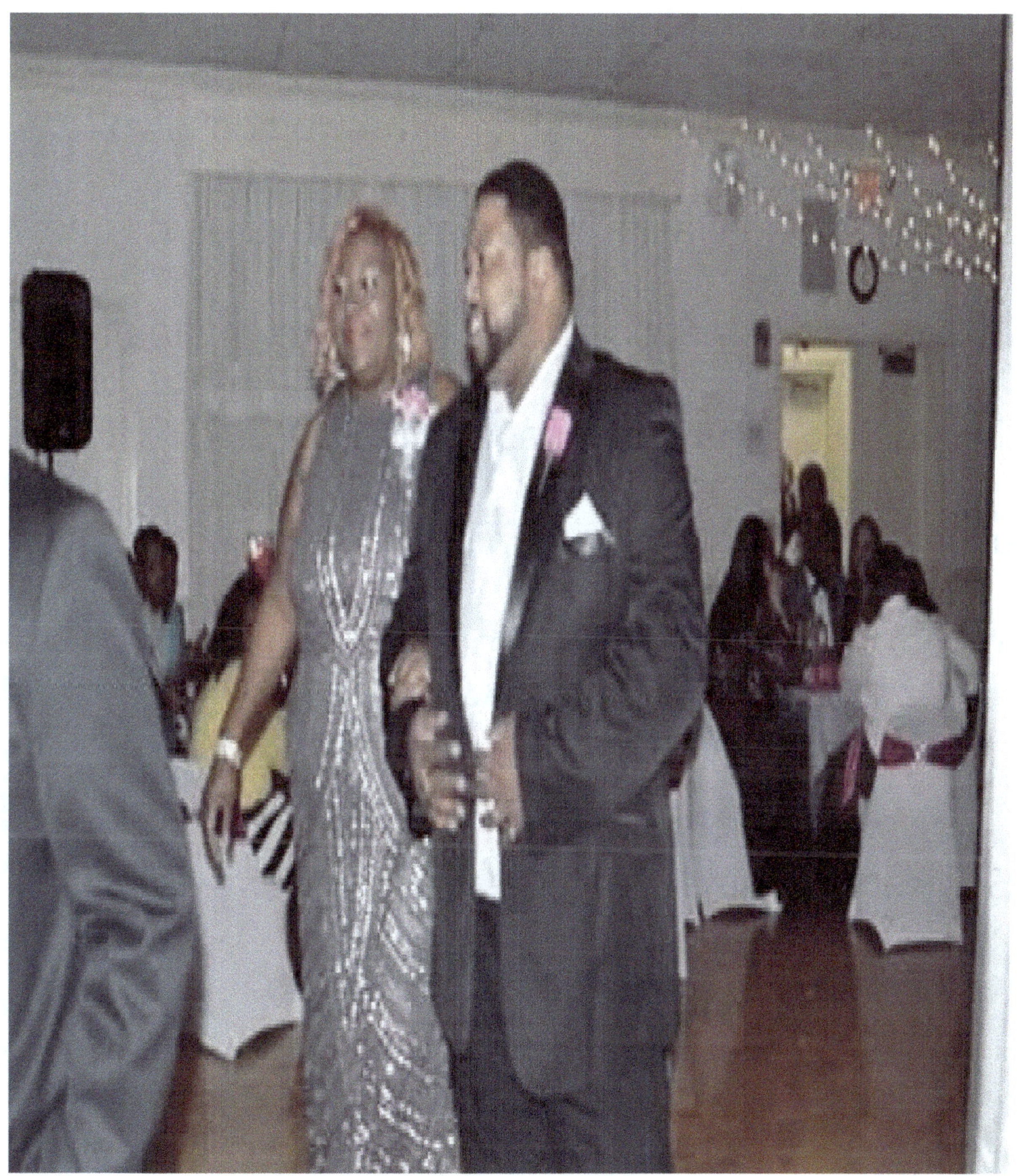

In my situation, I felt no other option was available to me because I put my body through so much. I couldn't exercise and just felt like I wouldn't live another year. I was at my breaking point, and I knew if I didn't do something fast, I would put my family through a painful unnecessary heart break. A little unselfishness is the word I finally realize how important I am to my loved ones.

Some days I didn't leave my bed until one day my wife gave me a message from God. She said, "Baby you must get out of the bed, the doctors have done all they can do, there's nothing left you are on every medication available. It's on you to get up out of that bed and do something about your health". It was then I decided to make some changes.

A few weeks after that message from my wife my oldest son James II had a talk with me, he said, "dad I'm not ready to have children, but I feel that when I do you won't be around for them. I want my kids to experience my dad, dancing, and saying crazy things, laughing". My heart dropped, tears came to my eyes, and I was more determined than ever to get my life

back.

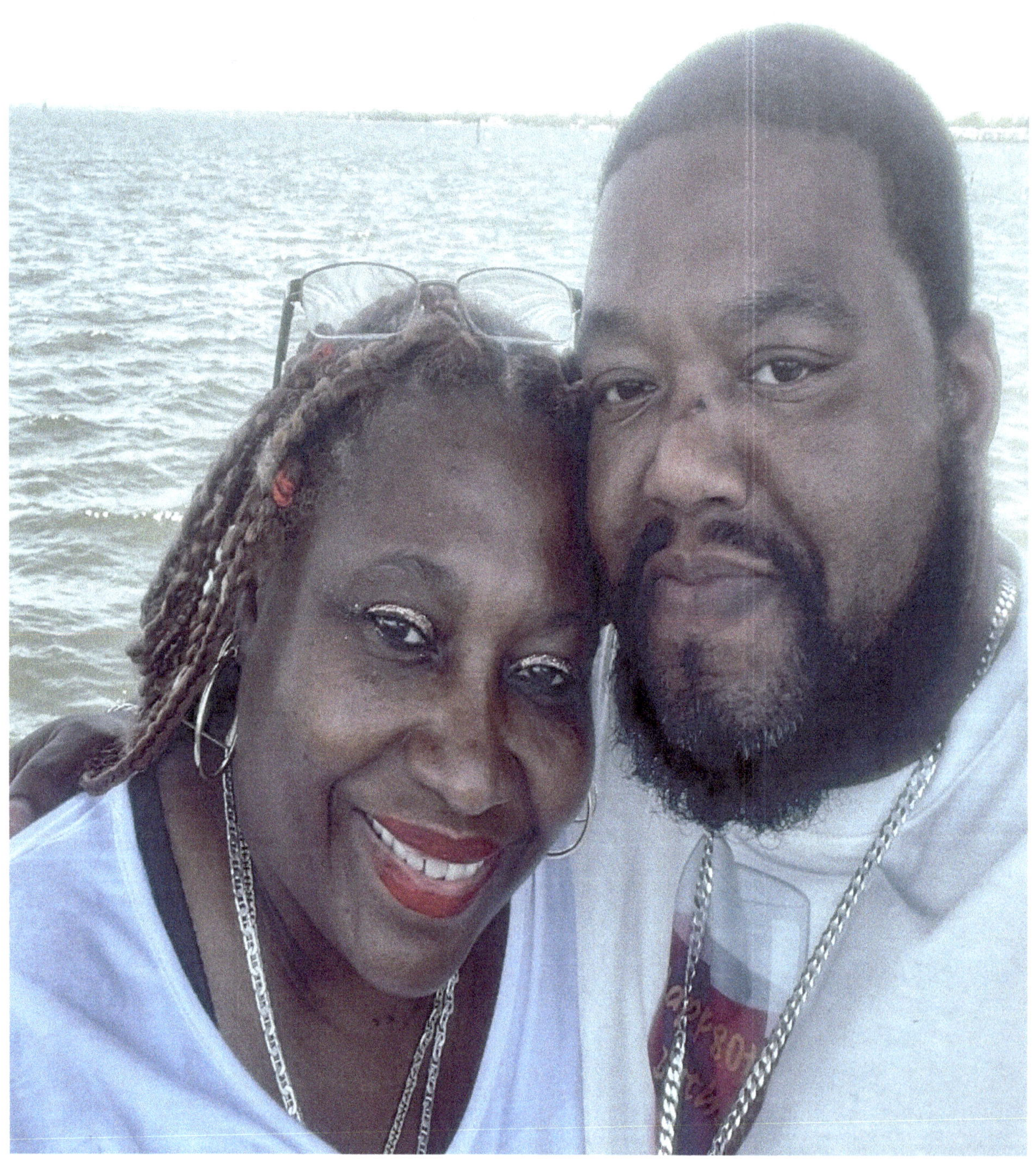

I started walking a little at a time, some days I felt ashamed as people seemed to look at me strange. I could imagine what they were saying {This fat man walks every day and still fat} I didn't let my feeling get in the way. So, I pushed forward determined to get my life back. I'd pushed myself which led to an unfortunate incident. I was saddened, when you really want something, life will give you many reasons to quit.

During my process I had many setbacks, people would say the devil is always busy! I had a finger issue that needed surgery. I truly feel that during that time when I was having the surgery, they moved me wrong because when I woke up my finger didn't hurt but my back and leg was giving me pain that was unbearable. Trying to get healthy now I would make a big mistake?

The doctors convinced me that I needed back surgery, I didn't know what to do but I knew I couldn't live with this pain, so I had the surgery. The surgery was unsuccessful as weeks went by, I was not feeling better, so I toke an MRI this reviled that the disc was re-herniated! I didn't do any activities to cause this the doctor said oh you can cough and re-herniate your disc.

I was angry but undeterred I pushed forward. After my back was healed from the incision I got up and out the house, in pain and continued my walks, in serious pain I pushed forward. Time went on and I was getting nowhere. I've thought about bariatric surgery in the past but never went deep in the process. This time was different I was not just thinking of myself and my fears.

I had my family in my heart, and they expressed the love they had for me and how important it was for me to live. The bariatric process was rough but if I had to do it again today I absolutely would, I feel amazing from sunup to sundown.

I have some days when I must deal with issues from the surgery but, they are minor compared to where I came from. If it wasn't for my back pain, I would be

100% but you can guarantee there will be no more

back surgeries in the future for me.

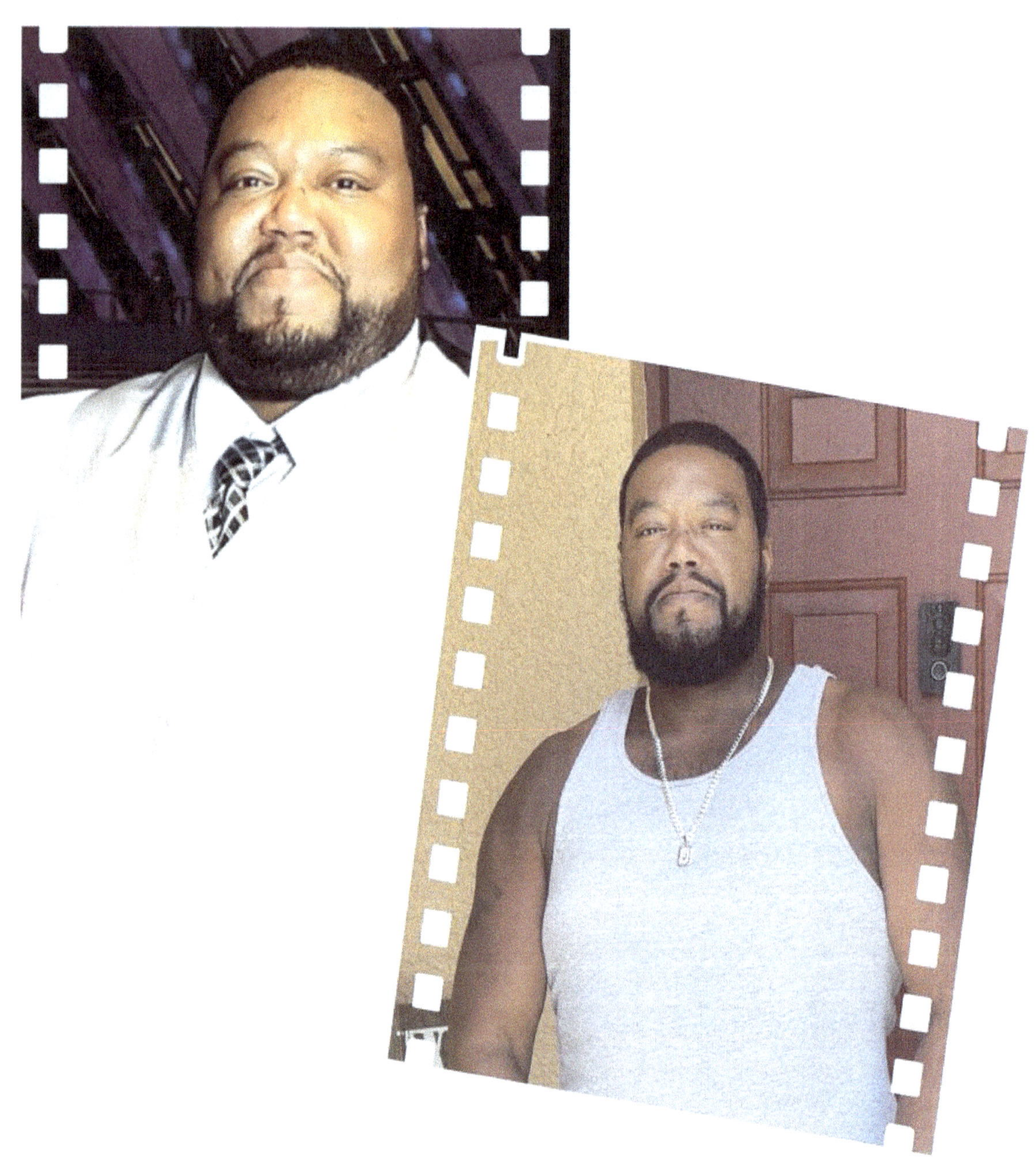

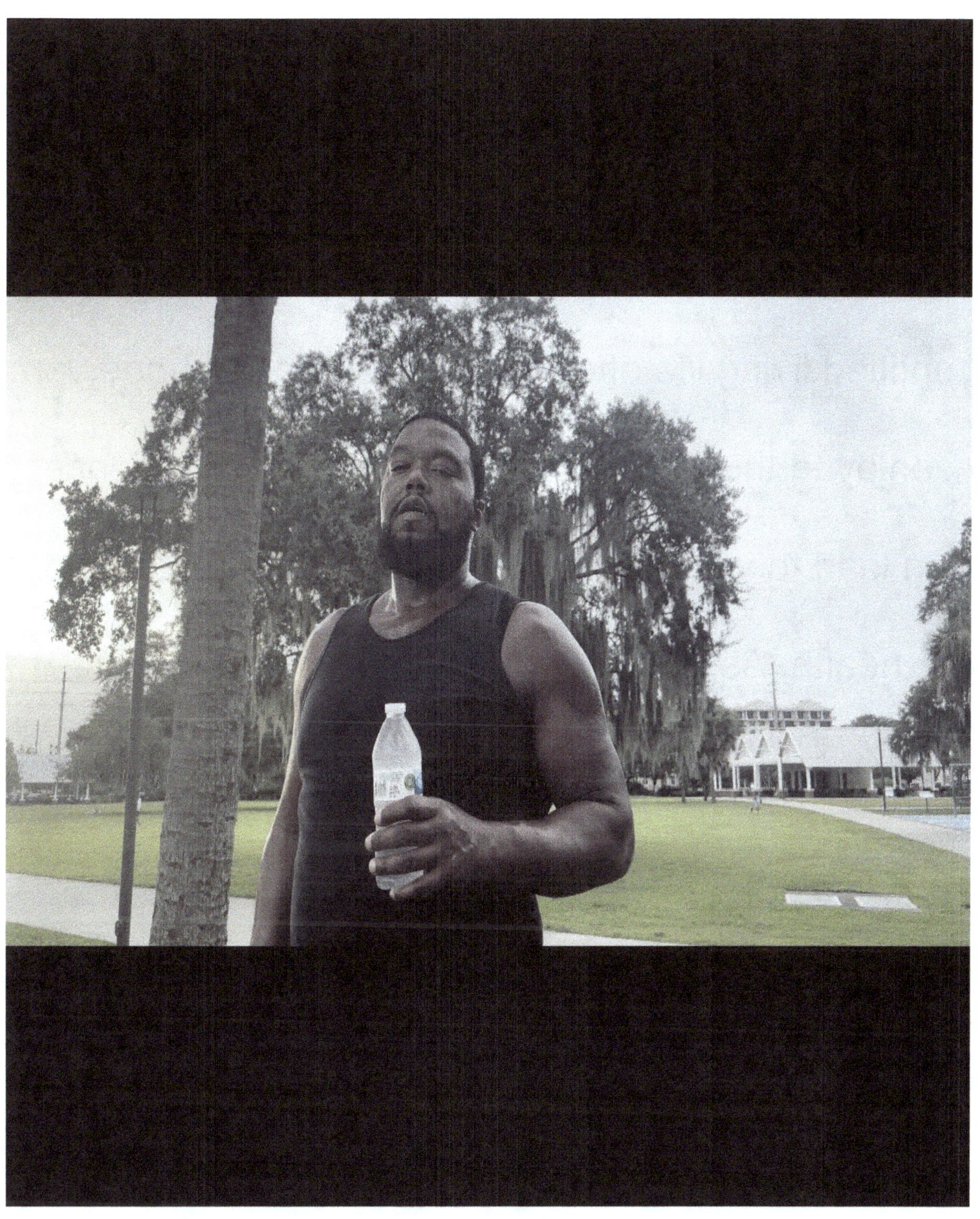

In one year, I will be completing my second book entitled living life after Bariatric Surgery. I hope you enjoyed this book and I hope that my experience can lead to your success in your path to restore your health. As always may God bless you, Amen.

Author James Kearney

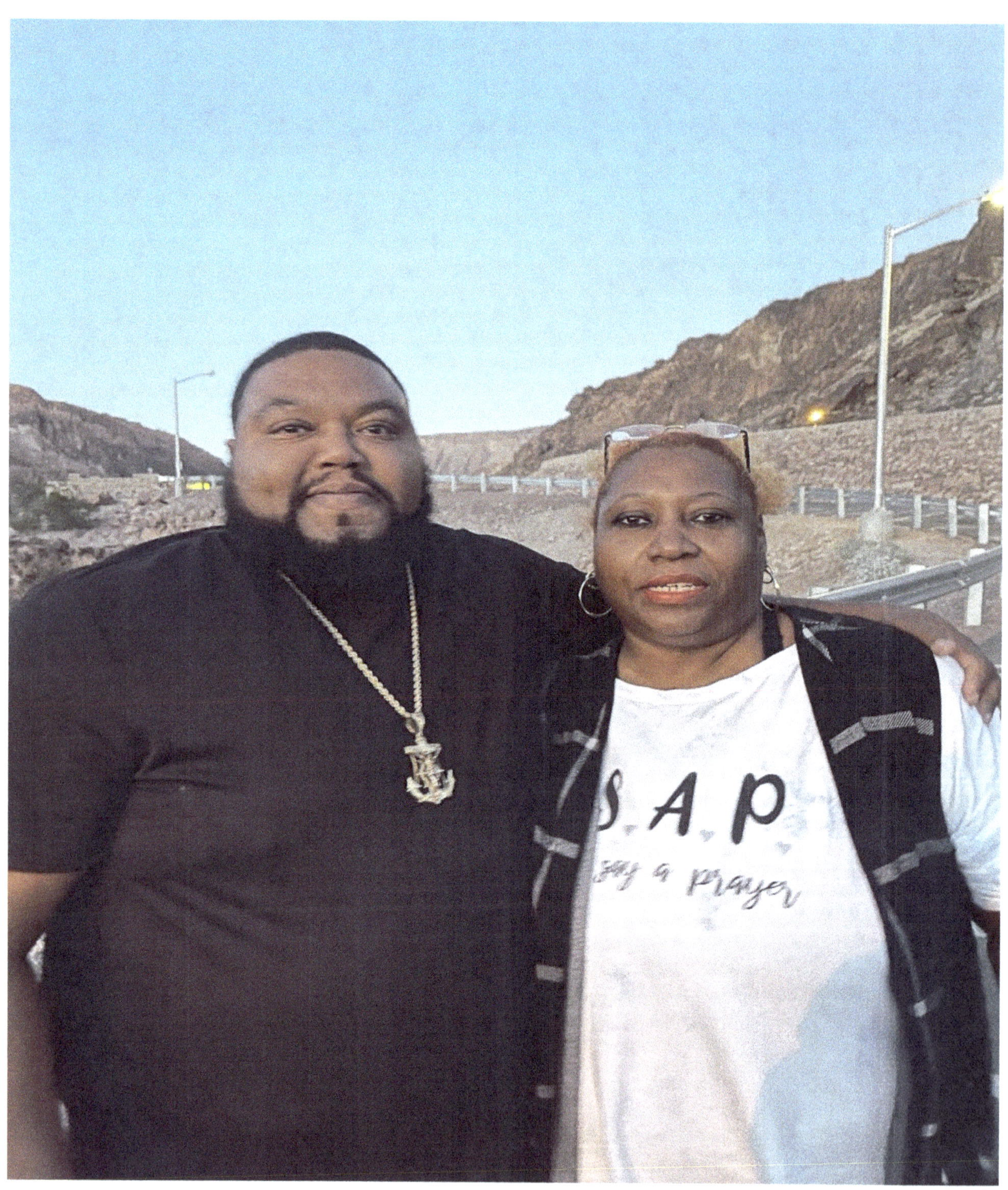
S.A.P
Say a prayer

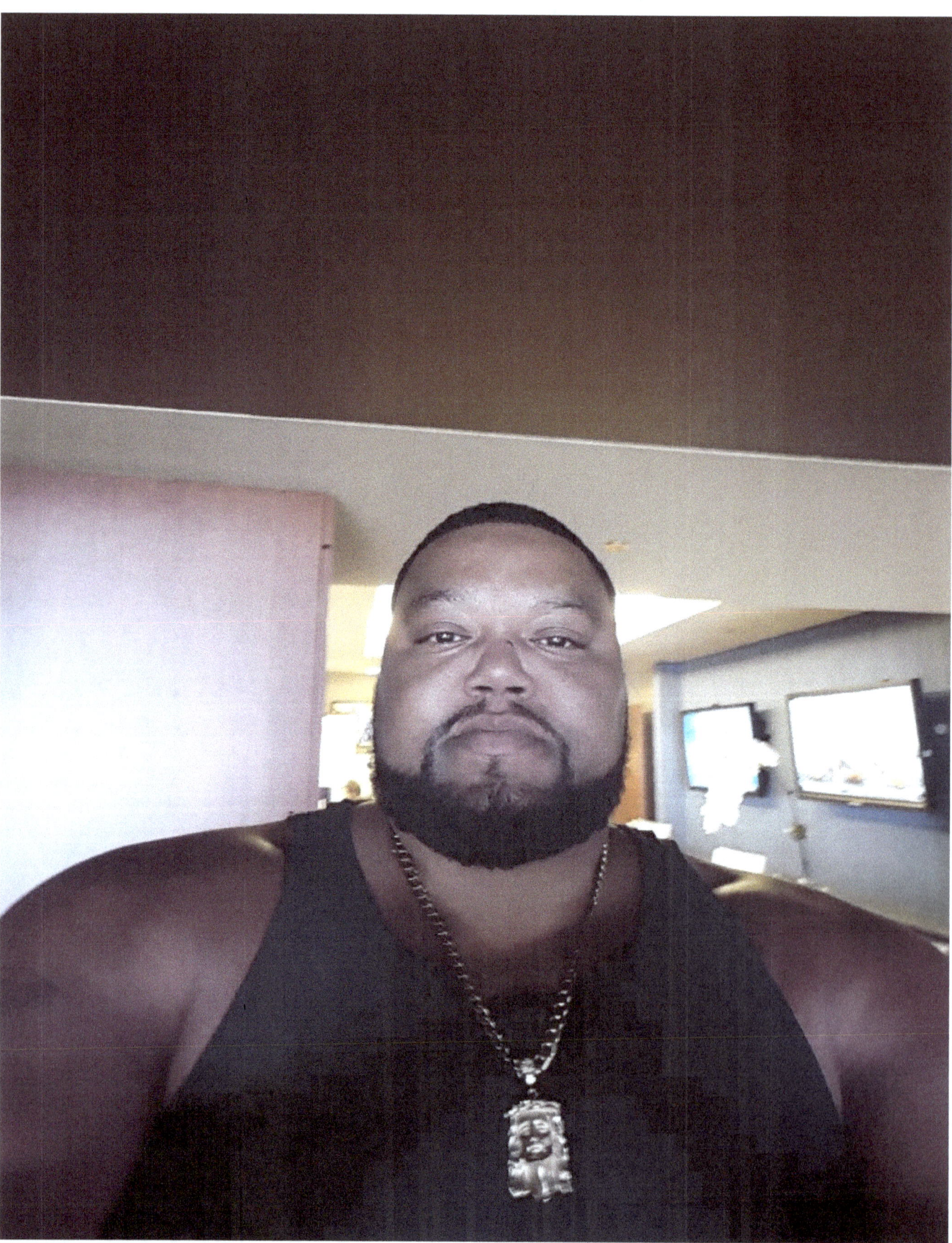

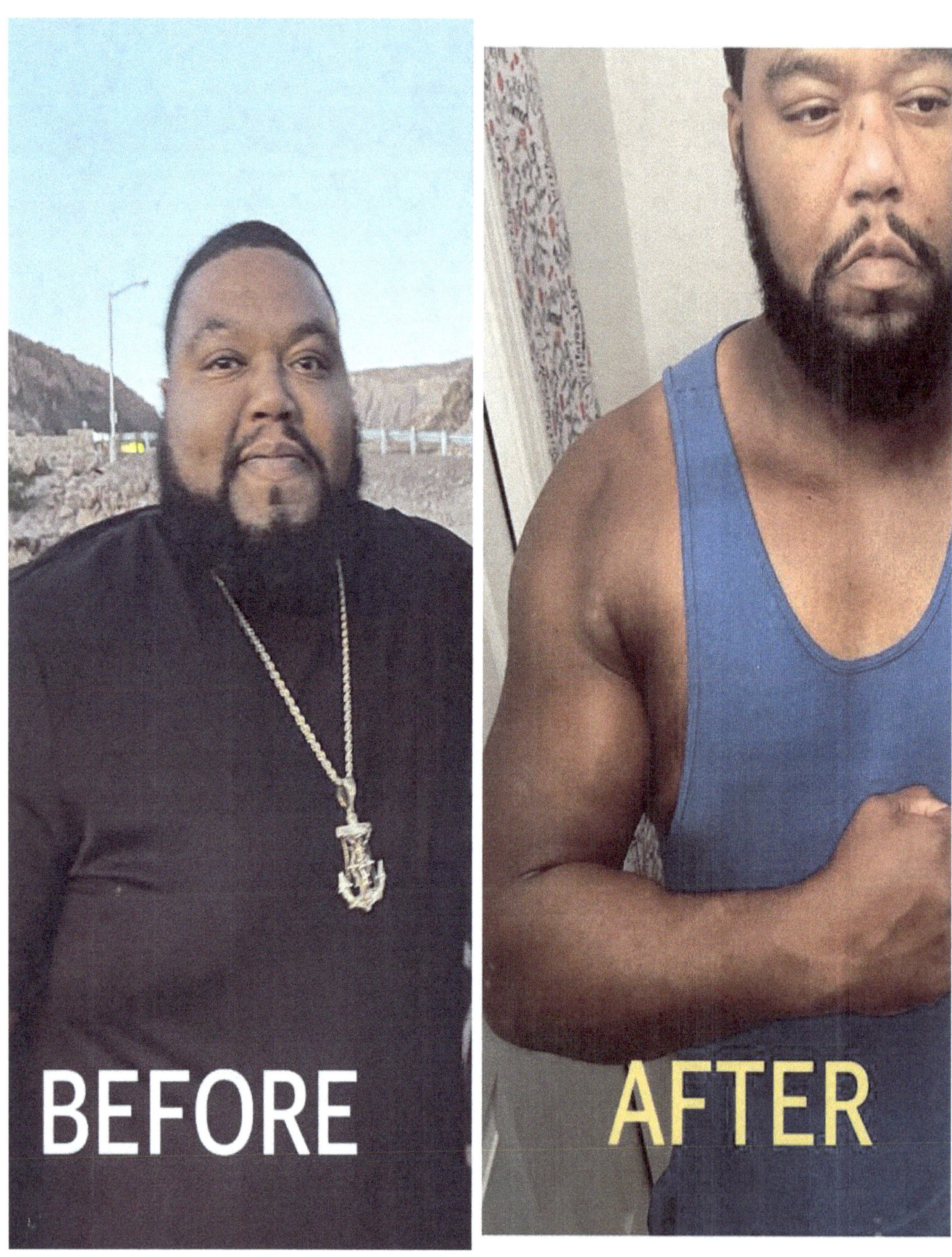

BEFORE
AFTER

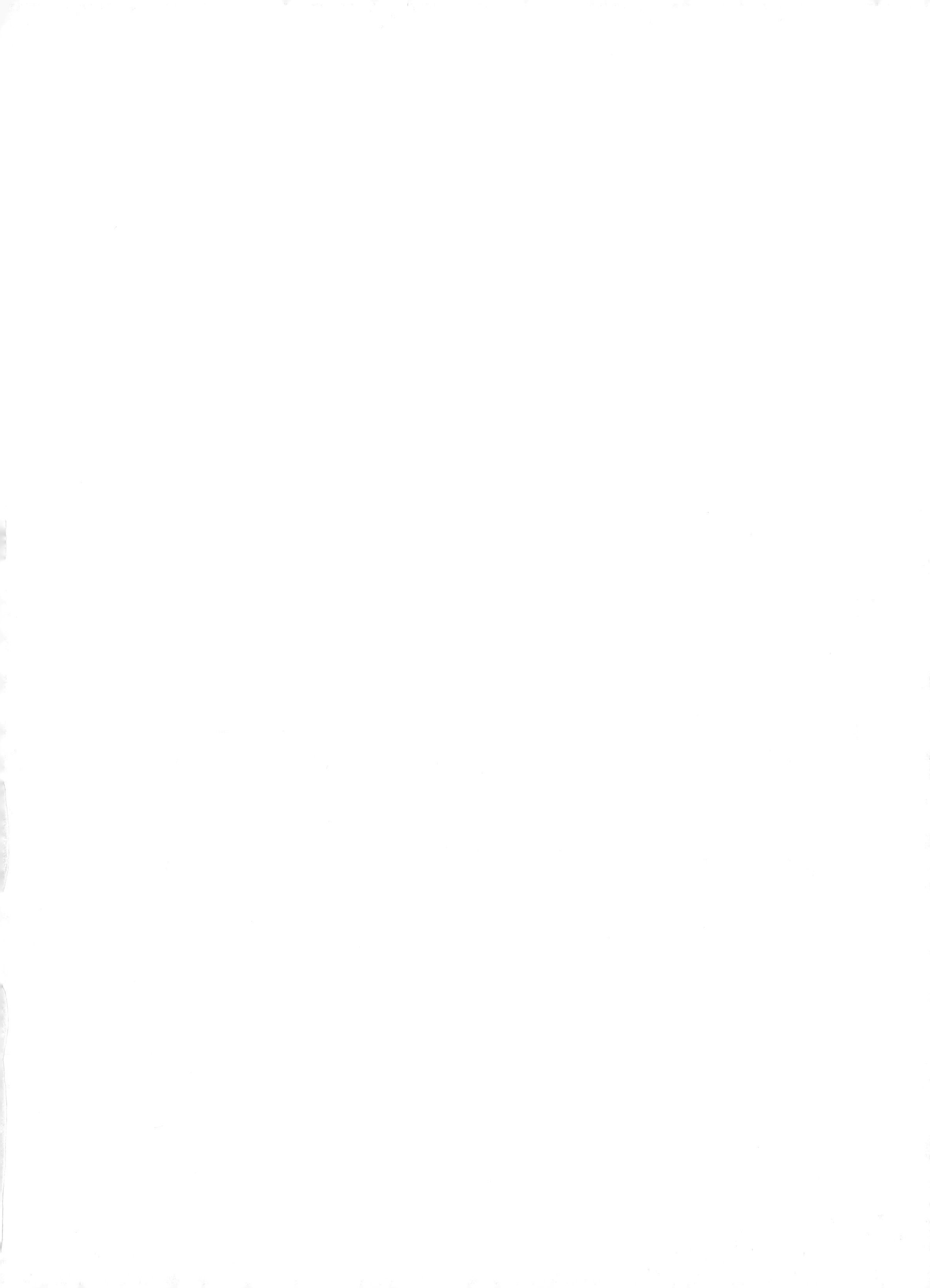